The Complete
Guide to
BREAST
CANCER

The Complete Guide to

BREAST CANCER

How to Feel Empowered and Take Control

Professor Trisha Greenhalgh and
Dr Liz O'Riordan

LONDON

1 3 5 7 9 10 8 6 4 2

Vermilion, an imprint of Ebury Publishing,
20 Vauxhall Bridge Road,
London SW1V 2SA

Vermilion is part of the Penguin Random House group of companies
whose addresses can be found at global.penguinrandomhouse.com

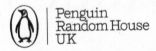

Copyright © Trisha Greenhalgh & Liz O'Riordan 2018

Trisha Greenhalgh and Liz O'Riordan have asserted their rights
to be identified as the authors of this Work in accordance with
the Copyright, Designs and Patents Act 1988

First published by Vermilion in 2018

www.penguin.co.uk

A CIP catalogue record for this book is available from the British Library

ISBN 9781785041877

Typeset in 11/15 pt Sabon LT Std
by Integra Software Services Pvt. Ltd, Pondicherry

Printed and bound in Great Britain by Clays Ltd, Elcograf S.p.A.

Penguin Random House is committed to a sustainable future
for our business, our readers and our planet. This book is
made from Forest Stewardship Council® certified paper.

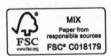

CONTENTS

ACKNOWLEDGEMENTS

We are grateful to the many people (too numerous to list here individually) who helped us through our own experiences of breast cancer and supported us in writing this book. The doctors and nurses who looked after us were outstanding in every way. They literally saved our lives.

Our families and friends (including those on social media) gave us practical help, companionship, common sense and humour when we needed it most.

Many people, acknowledged in the different chapters, gave permission to reproduce diagrams or other resources.

Clare Hulton, our agent, believed in this book from the outset and worked hard to find us the right publisher.

Sam Jackson and her team at Penguin Random House provided us with top-quality design, editing, proofreading and marketing support.

Most of all, our husbands (Dermot O'Riordan and Fraser Macfarlane) have been with us every step of the way and have never wavered in their love and support.

CHAPTER 1

JOINING THE CANCER CLUB

WE'VE BEEN THERE.

The moment you find out that you have breast cancer, your life changes forever. Your first reaction is likely to be one of shock, horror or disbelief. You may worry about what the future holds, and whether you will live long enough to see it. Most people who get breast cancer in the UK go on to live for many years and most do not die of breast cancer, but some will get a recurrence. However long you live for, you will never return to being a non-cancer patient.

For the rest of your life, you will be in one of two phases:

1. *Having active treatment.* This will include some or all of surgery, radiotherapy, chemotherapy, hormone therapy and other targeted therapies.
2. *Living after active treatment.* This is sometimes known as 'survivorship'. Your life will be interrupted by periodic hospital appointments, mammograms or scans, adjusting to the side effects of breast cancer treatment and coping with the possibility that your cancer might come back.

If your cancer comes back – called 'secondary cancer' – you enter a third phase, and this can happen even 20 years after your first diagnosis. This can, of course, be very upsetting, and we cover this in detail in Chapter 23 (page 256).

The first couple of weeks after diagnosis can be a period of uncertainty and confusion. You have to deal with the fact that you have got breast cancer, as well as taking in a lot of information about the treatments you need. Friends and relatives may ask you a lot of questions that you don't yet know the answers to. It can be hard to believe you have cancer because you don't feel (or look) ill. This is because, unless you have secondary breast cancer, the only symptom you are likely to have is a lump (and some people don't even have that). Unlike some other kinds of cancer, early breast cancer doesn't make you feel tired or short of breath or generally unwell.

WHY ME?

This is often the first question that people ask. The important thing to remember is that getting breast cancer is *not your fault*. The two biggest reasons why women get breast cancer are simply because they are women, and are getting older. Most breast cancers happen in women over the age of 50. Your breasts are made up of glandular tissue and fatty tissue. If your breasts have more glandular tissue than fat (known as 'dense breasts'), this can also increase your risk. All of these things are outside of your control. In a nutshell, most breast cancers are sensitive to the female hormone oestrogen, and the older you are, the more oestrogen you have been exposed to in your lifetime. The lifetime risk of a woman developing breast cancer is 1 in 8. While you are in your twenties, your risk of developing breast cancer is very small (1 in 2,000 women). During your sixties, your risk is higher (1 in 15 women).

There are other lifestyle factors that have been proven to increase the risk of developing breast cancer, and these include: being over-weight, not exercising regularly and drinking alcohol (more than the recommended guidance of two units a day), especially if you are post-menopausal. That being said, you can still get breast cancer if you are slim and exercise regularly, like we did.

There are other things that have been shown to increase the risk of breast cancer, such as taking the oral contraceptive pill or hormone replacement therapy (HRT) for many years, not breast-feeding your children or not having children at all. However, there is no way to prove that the reason you have breast cancer is because (for example) you took the pill when you were younger. For most of us, it is just bad luck, and again, it is not our fault. Men get breast cancer too, although this is rare (the lifetime risk of a man developing breast cancer is 1 in 870). We have written a separate chapter (Chapter 20, page 244) specifically for men with breast cancer.

A very small proportion of breast cancers, around 5 in every 100 cases, are linked to a strong family history of breast cancer, in which an altered ('mutated') gene is passed from a parent to a child. The most well-known mutations are in the BRCA1 and BRCA2 genes. An altered BRCA gene means that you have a 60–80 per cent chance of developing breast cancer and a 10–60 per cent chance of developing ovarian cancer in your lifetime. Other rarer genetic mutations include the TP53 gene and conditions like Peutz-Jegher syndrome and Cowden's syndrome. If several people on one side of your family have had breast or ovarian cancer below the age of 50, the altered gene might run in your family. Your GP or surgeon will be able to advise you whether you might be eligible for a gene test following genetic counselling. A full account of BRCA testing and what it involves is beyond the scope of this book, but the charity website Breast Cancer Care (www.breastcancercare.org.uk) is a good place to start looking for accurate information.

INFORMATION GATHERING

On the day you are diagnosed, you will know very little about your own breast cancer. You may have seen family or friends go through treatment, but they are not you. Even if you have done a lot of reading beforehand, have looked after people with breast cancer or are a medical expert in breast cancer yourself (like Liz was), you have never been a breast cancer patient before. And that is a completely different ball game.

At this stage, you may just want to sit back, go with the flow and let your medical team treat you without asking many questions. However, you may want to find out everything you can about breast cancer. You probably don't even know where (or what) to start reading – or what (if anything) to start worrying about. Even if you do not actively seek out information, you will soon become an expert in how *you* feel, how *you* react to good and bad news, and how *your* body tolerates different drugs and procedures. In that sense, most breast cancer patients become 'experts' within a few months of their diagnosis.

WHY WE WROTE THIS BOOK

We are both doctors – Trish is a GP and Liz is a breast cancer surgeon. We met on Twitter in July 2015 and became 'virtual chemo buddies' for breast cancer treatment, which we began (in different towns) in the same week. We first met in person six months later, which is when we had the idea for this book.

Between us we have had almost every kind of breast cancer treatment. Because we have both had breast cancer, we know, broadly speaking, what you are going through right now. And while we do not know exactly what *your own* personal circumstances are, we know what it's like to have your world collapse around you the moment you get your diagnosis, leaving you feeling powerless and alone.

But you are not alone. We wrote this book because we want to help people with breast cancer. This is the book we wish we had been able to buy the day we were diagnosed. Doctors tell you what will happen to you, but it is patients who will show you how to cope. We want to walk you through breast cancer, from beginning to end, and share the tips and tricks that helped us cope, both mentally and physically. We explain the main treatments that you will be offered, why they are being recommended to you and how they might make you feel. We talk about body image, relationships and sex, and how to stay healthy when treatment ends. We hope this book will serve as a companion and a guide to what is coming over the new few weeks, months and years.

There are many sources of information about breast cancer – including websites, books, blogs and newspaper articles. This book is not intended to replace all the other information out there. Indeed, it can be incredibly helpful to browse the websites of different cancer charities and to read patient blogs to get a real-life account of what a certain treatment might be like (see Liz's blog – liz.oriordan.co.uk – or simply search online for 'breast cancer blog'). However, sometimes it feels like there's too much information rather than not enough and it's important to bear in mind that not all of the information you will come across is accurate, and some of it may be very scary.

This book is intended to complement your own exploration of the information out there. We suggest you use it as a map to guide you at the different stages in your journey. It would be impossible to cover everything, but we hope you can dip in and out and get most of the information you need in the beginning.

Before we start, here are our own breast cancer stories. A lot of the words we use to describe our cancers and the treatment we had may seem foreign at the moment, but later in the book we will explain what all the terms mean.

Trish's story

In 2015 I was 56 and working part-time as a GP, but my main job was as a professor doing research and teaching at the University of Oxford. I work in a field called 'evidence-based medicine', which seeks to ensure that the tests and treatments offered to patients are informed by scientific research evidence. I have a husband, Fraser, and two grown-up sons, Rob and Al, who were 26 and 23 at the time of my diagnosis.

In May 2015, I noticed blood in my bra, and realised that my left nipple had been itching and flaky for several weeks. All my previous screening mammograms had been normal. I was seen in the breast clinic and my surgeon thought it might be eczema. The mammogram showed some calcification near the nipple, and the ultrasound was normal. I had a nipple biopsy on the same day which found some 'atypical' cells, but no evidence of cancer.

Because of the calcification on the mammogram, I was called back three weeks later for an X-ray-guided vacuum biopsy of the calcifications. That biopsy found both ductal carcinoma in situ (DCIS) and invasive breast cancer. The receptor status was ER-negative, PR-negative and HER2-positive. I was treated privately because I had insurance. I had a mastectomy, implant reconstruction with a tissue expander and a sentinel node biopsy. The final pathology report described 2.7cm of ductal carcinoma in situ (DCIS) and a tiny 0.8cm grade 2, Stage 1 invasive ductal carcinoma, along with Paget's disease of the nipple.

The total time from first being told I had breast cancer to getting my results after surgery was four weeks, but it seemed much longer! The good news was that my cancer was small and had not spread. The less good news was that, because my cancer was HER2-positive (a kind of cancer that can be aggressive), I needed to have chemotherapy and Herceptin treatment.

Ten days after my mastectomy, I started a three-month course of weekly chemotherapy with paclitaxel (Taxol). I wore a 'cold cap' which stopped my hair falling out. I had Herceptin injections every three weeks for a year, and my temporary implant was replaced with a permanent implant after I had finished chemotherapy. I also had two hospital admissions with a severe infection because chemo and Herceptin had lowered my immunity.

I felt generally rotten during chemo but managed to work (mostly from home) writing academic papers throughout this period. Getting back to all my duties at the university took many months – partly because of fatigue and partly because I kept getting coughs and colds. I was reluctant to return to work as a GP until I was fighting fit (since doctors can catch infections from their patients) and, as it turned out, I never did return to practising as a doctor, though this is mainly because my university job now keeps me fully occupied.

Liz's story

I'm a consultant breast cancer surgeon and spend my working life treating patients with breast cancer. My husband, Dermot, is also a surgeon. In July 2015, at the age of 40, I noticed a lump in my left breast. The mammogram was normal, but the ultrasound showed a suspicious 2.5-cm lump. The core biopsy showed a mixed ductal and lobular cancer which was ER-positive, PR-positive and HER2-negative.

Because my breasts were dense, I had an MRI scan. This showed that my cancer was actually closer to 6cm, which is often the case with lobular cancers as they can be hard to see on mammograms and ultrasounds. Within a week I started chemotherapy, which I can only describe as the worst hangover of my life without the dancing-on-tables-telling-the-world-you-love-them first. Chemo also threw me in to an instant menopause, which I really struggled with. My cancer shrank during chemo, and my last MRI showed that the cancer had actually disappeared.

I then had a mastectomy, implant reconstruction and a sentinel node biopsy. Two weeks later, just before Christmas, I learned that my cancer hadn't disappeared. There was 13-cm of residual lobular cancer in my breast. The cancer had also spread to two of my lymph nodes. I had further surgery to remove more lymph nodes then a three-week course of radiotherapy and was started on tamoxifen for ten years. I developed chronic post-mastectomy pain syndrome, and my implant developed a hard painful capsule because of the radiotherapy, which I had replaced through another operation to try and help with the pain.

My treatment took nine months in total, and it took me a good six to eight months to get my energy levels back to a place where I could even think about operating and seeing patients again. In May 2018, I was diagnosed with a local recurrence in my armpit. I had surgery to remove this, followed by more radiotherapy and an operation to remove my ovaries so that I could switch to letro-zole tablets.

CHAPTER 2

BREAST CANCER: AN OVERVIEW

BY LEARNING WHAT a breast is and how breast cancer develops, it will be easier to understand why and how your doctors are treating your cancer.

WHAT IS BREAST CANCER?

The breast sits on top of your main chest muscle (pectoralis major) and is the organ that produces milk after a woman has given birth. Your breast is shaped like a tear drop, with the tail extending towards your armpit. It is made up of lobules which contain milk-producing glands. These glands are connected by ducts which carry milk to the nipple. The ducts and lobules are surrounded by fat and connective tissue which give the breast its shape.

The breast has a network of blood vessels which supply nutrients and oxygen to the tissue, and a network of lymph vessels which drain fluid and waste products from the breast. The lymph vessels are connected to the lymph nodes (also known as glands) in your armpit.

Cells are the building blocks of your body. They divide to make more cells so your body can grow, heal and repair itself. All cells in the body have a series of checkpoints to identify and destroy abnormal cells. Cancer happens when a cell starts to grow in an uncontrolled fashion as a result of changes (mutations) in its genetic make-up which damage the normal checkpoints. This cancerous cell can now divide without restrictions, form a mass called a tumour or a cancer, and move around the body.

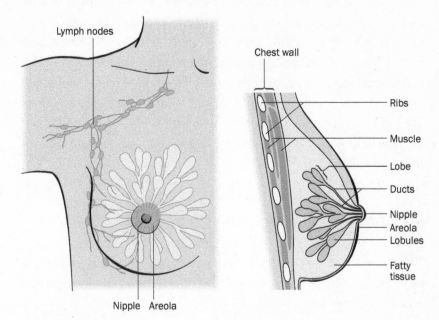

Lymph nodes

Chest wall

Ribs

Muscle

Lobe

Ducts

Nipple

Areola

Lobules

Fatty tissue

Nipple Areola

The female breast

Breast cancers develop from the cells in the ducts, lobules and connective tissue of the breast. Breast cancer first spreads through the lymph vessels to lymph nodes. The first lymph node in your armpit that your cancer spreads to is called the sentinel node. Breast cancers are normally slow-growing (although there are exceptions), and it can take several years for one cancerous cell to become a mass that can be seen on a mammogram or that you can feel.

Initially, breast cancer cells don't have the ability to move around the body and 'invade' your lymph nodes or other organs. These cancers are called 'non-invasive' (ductal carcinoma in situ or DCIS). Once the cells have developed the ability to spread, the cancer is called an 'invasive' breast cancer. (We explain these terms in more detail on 12–14.)

If you have primary breast cancer it means that your breast cancer hasn't spread beyond the lymph nodes in your armpit, is treatable and can potentially be cured. Sometimes your cancer can come back in your breast, the surrounding skin or your chest wall, called a 'local' recurrence. Alternatively, your cancer may spread to your bones or organs, such as your liver, lungs or brain, and this 'distant recurrence' is known as secondary breast cancer (also called metastatic or advanced cancer). At the moment, there aren't any treatments that can cure a cancer that has spread, but there are lots of treatments that can slow down the spread, prolong your life and help with any symptoms you may have (see Chapter 23 for more on this).

SUSPECTING BREAST CANCER

There are three ways that breast cancer may be suspected. If any of them happen to you, you will be referred to your local breast unit for further tests.

Breast change

The most common change is finding a lump in your breast. However, you may notice a rash on your nipple or breast, thickening, puckering or dimpling of the skin, in-drawing of your nipple or bloody discharge from your nipple. You may also have felt a lump in your armpit. Very rarely, you may notice an ulcer on your breast which is caused by a breast cancer that has grown through the skin (called a 'fungating' cancer). If you have any of these changes, you should see your GP for an urgent referral to your breast unit.

Recall from breast screening

In the UK, women between the ages of 50 and 70 are invited to have a mammogram (breast X-ray) every three years through the National Breast Screening Programme. Your mammogram might show something that needs further investigation, and this can sometimes be an early breast cancer.

Other scans or tests

You may have had a scan or a test to investigate another medical problem which showed either a cancer in your breast, or evidence of secondary cancer, such as a broken bone or a nodule in your liver. It is uncommon to find breast cancer in this way.

DIAGNOSING BREAST CANCER

Breast cancer is diagnosed using a 'triple assessment': an examination by a doctor or nurse, imaging (X-rays and/or scans) of the breast and armpit, and a biopsy of any suspicious areas. These should all happen during your first visit to the breast unit, but sometimes your biopsy may have to be done a few days later.

Examination

You will be seen by a doctor or nurse in the clinic. They will ask you about any breast changes, your family history of breast and ovarian cancer, and any medical conditions you might have. They will then examine your breasts and armpits, and, if they are concerned, will arrange for you to have some scans.

Imaging

The standard tests are a mammogram and an ultrasound scan (abbreviated as 'USS') of any lump or area of concern. If you are younger than 40, mammograms are not routinely done and you may just have an ultrasound to start with; mammograms are hard to interpret in young women because their breasts are dense. If the radiologist sees a suspicious area in your breast, you will also have an ultrasound scan of your armpit to look at the lymph nodes.

Biopsy

A small tissue sample called a 'biopsy' (technically a 'core biopsy') will be taken of any suspicious area in your breast or armpit. This is normally done at the same time as your ultrasound. It doesn't take long to do, and a local anaesthetic is used to numb the area first. It may feel a little uncomfortable, but it shouldn't hurt (though areas closer to the nipple are more sensitive). If the suspicious area is seen only on a mammogram, your biopsy will be taken using a special mammogram machine. You may feel that the lump has got bigger after the biopsy. This is due to swelling and bruising in the breast and is quite normal. If you have a rash on your breast or nipple, your doctor may take a very small skin sample called a 'punch biopsy'. Your biopsy will be examined by a pathologist to find out what type of breast cancer you have (see Chapter 3, page 25).

After the core biopsy, you may have a small gel clip inserted into the cancer that can be seen on future scans. There are two reasons for doing this:

1. If your cancer can't be felt, the clip guides your surgeon during your operation (see page 76).
2. If you are having chemotherapy before surgery, your cancer can shrink and sometimes disappear. The clip will guide your surgeon, so they know which part of your breast to remove.

TYPES OF BREAST CANCER

Non-invasive breast cancer

Non-invasive breast cancer (ductal carcinoma in situ or DCIS) develops in the cells of the breast ducts. This cancer does not have the ability to spread to other parts of your body. There are three grades (low, intermediate and high) which describe how close the DCIS is to becoming an invasive cancer. If DCIS isn't treated, it may develop into an invasive cancer in the months or years ahead. This is more likely to happen if your DCIS is intermediate- or high-grade, which is why surgery is recommended for it. At the time of writing, there are currently several trials investigating the treatment of low-grade DCIS to compare monitoring ('wait and see') with the standard surgical treatment, so national treatment guidelines for this kind of DCIS may change in the future.

Invasive breast cancer

Invasive breast cancer has the potential to spread to other areas of the body. There are several different types, depending on which cell in the breast the cancer has grown from:

Invasive ductal cancer

This accounts for 80 per cent of all breast cancers worldwide and develops from the breast ducts. It is also called NST (no special type) or NOS (not otherwise specified). It develops from cells in the milk ducts and is usually easy to see on a mammogram. There are some uncommon special types of invasive ductal cancer (tubular, medullary, mucinous, papillary and cribriform) that develop from specialised cells in the milk ducts. These are usually slow-growing and have an excellent prognosis. ('Prognosis' is an estimate of the likelihood that your cancer will come back. An excellent prognosis means that there is only a small chance that this will happen.)

Invasive lobular cancer

This accounts for 15 per cent of all breast cancers worldwide and develops from the breast lobules. It can be difficult to feel clinically and to see on a scan because the cells grow in sheets instead of forming a cluster like the invasive ductal cells. There are two types of lobular cancer. Classic lobular cancer is the most common type and is slow-growing. Pleomorphic lobular cancers are faster growing and can have a worse prognosis.

Invasive mixed cancer

This is a combination of ductal and lobular cancer cells and is usually treated like invasive ductal cancer.

Inflammatory breast cancer

This is a rare, aggressive form of breast cancer that looks like a breast infection (mastitis). Cancer cells block the lymph vessels in the breast and skin so the breast is warm, red and swollen.

Paget's disease of the nipple

This is a rare cancer that affects the cells of the nipple ducts, the surface of the nipple and the areola (the darker area around the nipple). The nipple develops a red and scaly rash which can become an ulcer and destroy the nipple. Most women with Paget's disease will also have DCIS, and some will have invasive breast cancer as well.

Phyllodes tumour

This is a very rare cancer that develops from the connective tissue in the breast. Most are benign (non-cancerous) but a small number can be malignant (cancerous). It rarely spreads to other parts of the body, and it is unlikely you will need any further treatment after your surgery.

WHAT HAPPENS IF YOUR DOCTOR CAN'T FIND YOUR BREAST CANCER?

If you notice a lump in your armpit and a core biopsy shows breast cancer cells, your surgeon will arrange for you to have a mammogram and ultrasound scan. Sometimes, these scans don't show a cancer in your breast. In this case, you will have an MRI scan, but sometimes this can also be normal. If the cancer in the breast can't be found, you will have surgery to remove your involved lymph nodes, with either a mastectomy or radiotherapy to the whole breast, probably followed by chemotherapy.

WHAT HAPPENS IF YOU HAVE SECONDARY BREAST CANCER WHEN YOU ARE DIAGNOSED?

In around 1 in 20 people with breast cancer, the cancer has already spread to other parts of the body when it is diagnosed (see Chapter 23). This may be devastating if it happens to you, and you and your doctors will have lots of decisions to make regarding how to treat your cancer. With primary cancer, the main treatment is surgery to remove the cancer. However, once your cancer has spread, the aims of treatment are to control the cancer (slow down or stop it spreading further), and to relieve any symptoms you have. This normally involves a combination of chemotherapy, hormone and targeted therapies, and most women have treatment for many months or years. Breast surgery itself becomes less important because the cancer has already spread, and your surgeon and oncologist will talk to you about whether you should have an operation.

PLANNING YOUR TREATMENT

In the UK, you have two treatment options. You can stay with the National Health Service (NHS) or have your treatment in the private sector (either through an insurance policy or paying your-self). If you're not already privately insured when you get breast cancer, you can't take out insurance to cover your treatment.

The NHS is fantastic when it comes to treating breast cancer. It has strict time targets so that everyone suspected of having cancer must be seen within two weeks. Your GP normally refers you to your local breast unit, but you can ask to be sent to a different hospital if you prefer. One of the breast team will see you, and you will be allocated to whichever surgeon is working in the hospital on the day you get your results. A different surgeon may then do your operation, together with his or her trainees. The NHS is a teaching environment, and junior surgeons will be supervised by your consultant while they perform certain parts of your operation. If you do want to be seen by a specific surgeon you can ask to see them personally, but it's not always possible (for example, they may be on holiday). Once you've been diag-nosed with cancer, it is recommended that you start your cancer treatment within 31 days from your diagnosis, whether this is surgery or chemotherapy.

Although the NHS is great, there are some benefits to private treatment:

- You can choose which surgeon you see.
- You will get more time with your surgeon in clinic appointments.
- You will probably get a nicer room in hospital.

However, it can be hard to know which surgeon to choose. If you wish to have your treatment privately, look at private hospital websites. Your GP may be able to recommend a private surgeon, and you can always ask your NHS surgeon whether they do private work.

Having private treatment should not change which treatments you have. Every breast surgeon should follow the same national guidance (see Chapter 6), whether they are working in the NHS or the private sector. If a private surgeon is offering you something radically different from what you'd get on the NHS, you should be wary. Private doctors are not as closely scrutinised as those in the NHS. If in doubt, discuss things with your GP.

> Liz had all her treatment on the NHS, while Trish was treated privately through a personal insurance policy. The treatment Trish had privately was exactly the same as she would have had on the NHS, but she was reassured that her consultant surgeon would do her operation without trainees being involved. There were also some comfort advantages (she got a single room in the hospital and the chemotherapy unit had its own chef).

Breast cancer treatment is planned on an individual basis, because every patient is different. Below we introduce the different professionals and explain how they work together to plan and deliver your treatment.

The multidisciplinary cancer care team

If you have cancer treatment on the NHS, your case will be discussed with a team of doctors and nurses at a multidisciplinary team meeting (also called an 'MDT'). In the US, this team is called a 'Tumor Board'. The MDT makes sure that your diagnosis of breast cancer is accurate, agrees a treatment plan (taking into account your type and size of cancer, whether it has spread and your general health) using the latest evidence-based guidelines (explained in Chapter 3), and discusses any research trials that might be relevant to you (see Chapter 6). If you are being treated privately, your surgeon should use an MDT as well. The key people in an MDT include:

Breast surgeons and trainees

Breast surgeons are doctors who specialise in breast surgery. A consultant is the most senior surgeon who has finished all their specialist training.

Plastic surgeons

Plastic surgeons are surgeons who specialise in repairing or reconstructing missing tissue or skin, like a breast reconstruction. Your breast surgeon may work together with a plastic surgeon if you need a breast reconstruction (see Chapter 8). They normally only get involved in MDTs in larger hospitals, as most small hospitals don't have plastic surgeons on site.

Breast radiologists and radiographers

Breast radiologists are doctors who specialise in looking at breast and body scans. Radiographers are specially trained technicians who do mammograms and ultrasounds.

Breast pathologists

Breast pathologists are doctors who specialise in looking at breast tissue under the microscope and they write your pathology report (see Chapter 3).

Breast oncologists

Breast oncologists are doctors who specialise in treating primary and secondary breast cancer with chemotherapy, radiotherapy and Herceptin, and other targeted therapies. They will estimate your prognosis (see Chapter 3) and plan what extra treatment you need.

Radiotherapy specialists and radiotherapists

Radiotherapy specialists and radiotherapists are nurses and technicians who will give you information, help plan and deliver your treatment, and look after you during radiotherapy.

Specialist nurses

Breast care nurses and oncology nurses are specially trained to look after breast cancer patients. They work with the doctors in out-patient clinics and will look after you, give you information and offer emotional support. They are usually your first port of call if you have a problem and you should feel able to discuss any worries that you might have about your possible treatment plan with them.

MDT coordinator

The MDT coordinator makes sure that all the treatment plans agreed in the MDT are properly recorded, and that you have all your treatments promptly, according to the NHS cancer pathway targets (see Chapter 6). If you are having a second opinion, they will make sure that all your scans and reports have been sent from your first hospital.

It normally takes a week or two from the date of your biopsy for your results to be processed and discussed at the MDT. Sometimes, you may need to have further tests or biopsies before you can be treated. This could be another ultrasound scan to look at a different area in the breast, or an MRI scan. MRI scans are not done routinely, but may be needed if you have lobular cancer, very dense breasts or have cancer in your lymph nodes but no visible cancer on a mammogram (this is called an occult cancer).

It can take several weeks for these extra scans and biopsies to be performed and analysed, and it is hard not to feel anxious that the cancer is spreading. Remember that it can take several years for a breast cancer to grow, and it is more important for your team to get all the information they need so you can have the correct treatment, instead of rushing ahead and possibly missing something important.

The primary healthcare team

One of the first things you should do after being diagnosed with breast cancer is make an appointment to see your general practitioner (GP). If you don't have a GP, or if the GP you do have is not someone you feel you can approach, now is the time to find a good GP local to you and re-register. To find one, see the excellent NHS Choices website: www.nhs.uk.

Your surgeon will send your GP a letter telling them about your diagnosis within a couple of days. Your GP can prescribe any medication that you need to take, advise on minor side effects and negotiate with the hospital on your behalf if needed. Incidentally, having cancer means you are eligible for free prescriptions in the UK, so ask your GP for the relevant form to fill in.

Your GP is not a cancer specialist, but they may be a (relative) expert on *you*. They know your other medical conditions, how you have reacted to serious illness in the past, your family circumstances and your wider support networks. A good GP is an 'active listener', able to hear your story and help you make sense of what's happening and help support your family. Some GPs are trained in cognitive behavioural therapy (CBT), which can help a lot if you need to deal with anxiety and negative thoughts (see page 40). Most GP practices often have nurse practitioners (highly trained nurses) who may see patients and prescribe drugs and give injections like Zoladex (see Chapter 13).

The final person to mention is your dentist. If you are going to need chemotherapy or bisphosphonates to strengthen your bones, try to get a check-up before you start, as your body won't tolerate drillings and fillings well during treatment.

Getting a second opinion

Before agreeing to your treatment plan, you may want to see a second surgeon to get a second opinion. Your GP should be able to refer you to another surgeon, or you may choose to see someone privately. Before you see them, you must think carefully about your reasons for getting a second opinion. Do you want someone to tell you what you want to hear, even if it means getting a third or a fourth opinion? Or do you want another sensible opinion, and if that's the same as your initial surgeon, will you then stick with the original treatment plan?

Everyone is entitled to a second opinion, but it could delay your cancer treatment. Your new surgeon must discuss your case in their own MDT which could take a week or two. In most cases, those extra couple of weeks will make no difference to your overall survival from breast cancer, but if getting your surgery as quickly as possible is your top priority, then getting a second opinion might not be in your best interests.

BREAST CANCER TREATMENT

We cover all of the treatments described below in detail in further chapters, but here is a brief summary of which treatments you might be advised to have:

Surgery

The main treatment for primary breast cancer is surgery (see Chapter 7). If you have invasive breast cancer, you will almost certainly be advised to have an operation to remove it. The two main operations are a lumpectomy (just the cancerous bit is removed) or a mastectomy (the whole breast is removed). If you need to have a mastectomy, your surgeon should discuss breast reconstruction with you (see Chapter 8).

You will also have an operation to remove one or more of the lymph nodes in your armpit – either a sentinel node biopsy or an axillary node clearance. If you only have DCIS, your cancer cannot spread to your lymph nodes, so you do not need to have your lymph nodes removed. The one exception is if you have a large area of DCIS and need to have a mastectomy – there is a small chance that you may have a small invasive cancer in your breast, and your surgeon will then remove a few lymph nodes at the same time as carrying out your mastectomy.

Chemotherapy

Chemotherapy is recommended if you have a high risk of developing secondary breast cancer in the future, and if you already have secondary breast cancer. It is normally given after surgery (adjuvant chemotherapy), but, as we will explain on page 132, your surgeon may recommend that you have it first (neoadjuvant chemotherapy). Chemotherapy drugs kill cells that are growing quickly, like cancer cells, but they also affect some of the normal cells in your body (see Chapter 10).

Targeted therapies

If your cancer is 'HER2-positive' (sometimes written as 'HER2+ve'), you will be offered a drug called Herceptin which will greatly improve your prognosis. At the time of writing, Herceptin has to be given with chemotherapy. You may be given other drugs that also target HER2+ve cancers. If you have secondary breast cancer, you may be given one of several other drugs that specifically target breast cancer cell growth (see Chapter 11 for more details).

Radiotherapy

Radiotherapy is used to reduce the risk of a local recurrence – when your cancer comes back in your breast or chest wall and lymph nodes (see Chapter 12). Everyone who has a lumpectomy needs to have radiotherapy to treat the breast tissue left behind. You may also need it after a mastectomy or if you have cancer in your lymph nodes. Radiotherapy is also used to treat symptoms of secondary breast cancer, and for pain control.

Hormone therapy

If your cancer is sensitive to oestrogen (ER-positive, usually written as 'ER+ve'), you will be given tablets to lower the levels of oestrogen in your blood and reduce the risk of your cancer returning in the future (see Chapter 13). If you are pre-menopausal, your oncologist may also discuss treatment to switch off your ovaries to further lower your oestrogen levels (see page 174).

Getting diagnosed with breast cancer can be very frightening, and you may feel like there is too much information to take on board. We know – we've been there. Once your diagnosis has started to sink in a little, one of your first questions may be, 'How long have I got?'. In the next chapter, we're going to tell you how your doctors estimate what your chances of surviving breast cancer are, and what additional treatments, on top of your surgery, you might need.

CHAPTER 3

LEARNING MORE

YOUR SURGEON WILL have a good idea of what treatment you need when they get the results of your core biopsy and your breast scans. However, they won't be able to give you more accurate information (such as whether you need chemotherapy or what your prognosis is) until after you have had your surgery. This chapter will help you to understand why your team is recommending certain treatments for your breast cancer, and how your outcome after treatment is estimated.

UNDERSTANDING YOUR PATHOLOGY REPORT

Your core biopsy (see page 12) gives your doctors a snapshot of your breast cancer, but it doesn't give them the full picture. Once your breast cancer and lymph nodes have been removed, a pathologist (see page 18) carefully analyses them. This gives your doctors all the details they need to help them plan what further treatment you need. You should be given most of this information to keep for your own personal records. The pathologist may refer to your breast cancer as a 'tumour'. Below are the different elements that are included in a typical report.

Tumour size

In most cases, your actual tumour size is very close to the size on your scans, but sometimes it can be much larger. The pathologist may also find other areas of cancer in your breast. These are described as 'multicentric' (when the cancers are in different areas) or 'multifocal' (when the cancers are close to each other, in the same area). If you have more than one area, only the size of the largest cancer is used to work out your prognosis. If you have an invasive cancer, the pathologist may also find non-invasive cancer. However, they only use the size of your invasive cancer to work out your prognosis.

Tumour type

This is usually the same as the cancer identified on your core biopsy, but sometimes a different type of cancer is also found. The different tumour types are described in Chapter 2 (pages 12–14).

Tumour grade

This is an indicator of how quickly your cancer cells are growing and how different they look compared to a normal breast cell. Invasive breast cancer has three grades: Grade 1 is slow-growing; Grade 2 cancer grows more quickly; and Grade 3 cancer grows faster still. DCIS also has three grades – low, intermediate and high – which refer to how quickly the cells are growing and how close to an invasive breast cancer they are.

Margin status

When your surgeon removes your breast cancer, they also need to remove a rim of normal breast tissue around it to make sure that no cancer cells are left behind. This rim is called a 'margin' (explained in more detail on page 77). There are six margins – those around the sides of the cancer (superior, medial, inferior and lateral); the anterior margin (between the cancer and your skin); and the posterior margin (between the cancer and your chest wall). The pathologist will record whether these margins are clear of cancer cells. If they are involved, you may need another small operation to remove more tissue at the involved margin.

Lymphovascular invasion

Lymphovascular invasion is when some of the cancer cells have invaded into neighbouring blood and lymph vessels. It means there is a greater chance that your cancer could spread to your lymph nodes or beyond.

Hormone receptor status

A hormone is a chemical messenger that controls the growth and activity of normal cells. Hormone receptors sit on the outside of cells and bind the hormone. Some breast cancer cells have receptors for the hormones oestrogen and progesterone, and the cancer depends on these hormones to grow. If your cancer has oestrogen receptors it is called ER-positive (ER+ve), and if it has progesterone receptors, it is called PR-positive (PR+ve). The oestrogen receptor results are more important when it comes to planning treatment, which involves lowering the levels of oestrogen in your body (see Chapter 13). If your cancer does not have these receptors it is called ER-negative (ER-ve) and PR-negative (PR-ve). If you have non-invasive cancer (DCIS), the hormone receptor status is not normally recorded because it doesn't affect your treatment plan.

HER2 receptor status

Every breast cancer cell produces a protein called Human Epidermal Growth Factor Receptor 2 (HER2). Around 15–20 per cent of breast cancers overall express very high levels of HER2, which cause the cancer to grow more quickly. If your cancer is HER2+ve, you will be offered treatments like Herceptin which specifically target HER2 (see Chapter 11). HER2 receptor status is not recorded for non-invasive cancer (DCIS). If your cancer is ER-ve, PR-ve and HER2-ve, it is known as a 'triple negative' cancer.

Lymph node status

The pathologist will look at your lymph nodes to see if they contain cancer cells. If there aren't any cancer cells, your lymph nodes are described as 'negative'. If there are cancer cells, your nodes are classified according to how much of the node is involved:

- Isolated tumour cells (ITCs): very small clusters of cells measuring less than 0.2mm.
- Micrometastasis: small deposit of cancer cells, measuring between 0.2mm and 2mm.
- Macrometatasis: large deposit of cancer cells, measuring more than 2mm.

Lymph nodes with ITCs or micrometastases are classed as negative. If your nodes are negative, you shouldn't need to have any further treatment. Lymph nodes with macrometastases are classed as positive. Extra-capsular spread means that the cancer cells have invaded beyond the wall of the node. If you have positive nodes, you may need to have further treatment such as surgery and/or radiotherapy. This depends on how many of your nodes are involved.

ASSESSING WHETHER YOUR CANCER HAS SPREAD

If you have DCIS or primary breast cancer that hasn't spread to your lymph nodes, it is very unlikely that you will have cancer elsewhere. However, if you do have cancer in your lymph nodes, there are some scans and blood tests that can be carried out to see whether your cancer has spread beyond the lymph nodes.

Staging scans

The National Institute for Health and Care Excellence guidelines (see page 64) recommend that only patients with large tumours or several involved lymph nodes should have extra scans to see whether their cancer has spread beyond the nodes. Most of the time, these scans are normal. It is rare for a scan to find distant disease in a patient without any symptoms of secondary cancer, such as bone pain or shortness of breath (see Chapter 23).

There are two scans that are routinely done:

1. A CT scan of your chest, abdomen and pelvis.
2. A bone scan.

Some hospitals use only a CT scan. It is important to understand that both of these scans cannot pick up individual cancer cells. A secondary deposit has to be large enough to show up, and this means that a normal CT or bone scan may still mean that there are sleeping cancer cells in your body. If you do get symptoms suspicious of recurrence in the future, your doctor may order scans to investigate further. The signs to look out for are detailed on pages 268 and 270.

Blood tests

At the moment, there aren't any blood tests that can accurately tell whether your cancer has spread or will spread in the future. If you have secondary breast cancer, your oncologist may measure tumour markers (proteins called CEA, CA15-3 and CA125). The results of these blood tests can vary greatly from patient to patient, depending on the amount of disease they have and the treatment they are having. If your staging scans are normal, you will not have routine tumour marker bloods taken on the NHS. You may have them done if you are being treated privately, but the value of such tests in people with early breast cancer is questionable.

PROGNOSIS IN BREAST CANCER

Prognosis is an estimate of the likelihood that your cancer will come back, and whether you will die from breast cancer. It is expressed in words (excellent, good, poor) or as a number (typically a percentage).

It reflects your 5- or 10-year survival rate, which is the likelihood that you will still be alive in 5 or 10 years' time. If your 10-year survival rate is 90 per cent, this means than out of 100 women that are the same age as you, with identical breast cancers and identical treatment, 90 of them will still be alive in 10 years' time. Your doctors will use your estimated prognosis to decide what further treatments you should have to reduce the risk of your cancer coming back.

Asking your doctor what your prognosis is can be scary, and finding out can be even scarier. It may all seem too much and you might not want to know. Your doctor will be guided by you, and should only tell you what you're ready to hear. If you do find out, you must remember that it is only an *estimate*. Your doctor has no way of knowing for certain whether your cancer will come back in the future.

Why is prognosis important?

Your doctor needs to know what your estimated prognosis is so they can decide whether to recommend other treatments such as chemotherapy. As we explain on page 31, not everybody needs chemotherapy, and not everybody who has chemotherapy will benefit from it.

The methods used to estimate your prognosis are based on large research trials that have looked at the survival of hundreds and thousands of people with breast cancer. In order to work out your chance of being alive in 10 years' time, these trials had to follow patients up for at least 10 years. This means that your actual prognosis may be *better* than your estimated prognosis, because new treatments are always being developed that improve your survival from breast cancer, but we don't yet have the 10-year follow-up data for those treatments.

Estimating your prognosis

The main factors used to work out your prognosis are your cancer type, size and grade, whether it has spread to your lymph nodes, whether it is sensitive to oestrogen (ER+ve) or Herceptin (HER2+ve), as well as your age and whether or not you have been through the menopause. Your doctor gets all this information from the pathology report (see page 24) after you have had your surgery, and they will be able to tell you what your prognosis is, if you want to hear it, when you go back to clinic to get your results after your operation.

Generally, small, low-grade, node-negative, ER+ve and HER2-ve cancers have a better prognosis than larger, higher grade, node-positive, triple negative and HER2+ve tumours. However, additional treatments, such as chemotherapy and Herceptin therapy, are given to improve the prognosis of these cancers. In fact, many people with a 'poor prognosis' cancer go on to live a long and heathy life. There are also things you can do to improve your prognosis, such as staying active and exercising, and we talk more about this in Chapter 18.

There are several methods used to estimate prognosis, and some are more accurate than others. None of them will tell you for sure whether the cancer will ever come back, but they will give you some idea of how likely that is:

Nottingham Prognostic Index (NPI)

This is a quick and simple calculation that uses the size of your cancer, its grade and the number of positive lymph nodes to give a rough estimate of your prognosis. Your NPI will either be excellent (below 2.4), intermediate (between 2.4 and 5.4) or poor (above 5.4).

Staging

Your breast cancer stage combines two things: how big your cancer is and whether it has spread. There are four stages which are each subdivided into several sub-stages, from Stage 1 (small with no or minimal spread to lymph nodes) to Stage 4 (secondary or metastatic breast cancer). The staging system is mainly used in America, where they have just introduced a new version which takes into account your hormone and HER2 receptor status. In the UK, your surgeon may use a similar system called 'TNM' (tumour size, number of positive nodes and presence of metastases).

If you are interested in the details of how to work out your stage, see the 'breast cancer stages' section of the Breast Cancer Care website: www.breastcancercare.org.uk/information-support/facing-breast-cancer/diagnosed-breast-cancer/diagnosis/breast-cancer-stages

Computer programs

For a more precise estimate of your prognosis, your doctor uses a mathematical model. In the UK, doctors tend to use PREDICT while in the USA, doctors tend to use Adjuvant! Online (see page 276). Both were developed by analysing the outcomes of thousands of women and then testing the data on thousands more.

PREDICT analyses the details of your cancer as well as your age and how your cancer was detected. It calculates your 5- and 10-year survival based on the following scenarios: surgery (and radiotherapy if needed), additional hormone therapy and additional chemotherapy (with Herceptin if your cancer is HER2+ve). You can use the PREDICT website yourself to see your own results: www.predict.nhs.uk

DECIDING WHETHER YOU NEED CHEMOTHERAPY

Only about a third of all patients with breast cancer are offered chemotherapy (see Chapter 10). Your doctor needs to weigh up the benefits (reducing your chance of developing, and dying from, secondary breast cancer) against the risks (serious side effects which can sometimes be permanent – and, very rarely, fatal).

Your doctors use your estimated prognosis to decide whether you are likely to benefit from chemotherapy. In the UK, doctors use your PREDICT results. Let's say, for example, that your PREDICT score gives you an estimated 10-year survival of

70 per cent with no further treatment, 80 per cent with hormone therapy and 90 per cent with chemotherapy as well. Would you take a punt on chemo with these odds? Most people would, since chemo could increase your chance of being alive in 10 years' time from 80 per cent to 90 per cent – a 10 per cent absolute improvement. If the figures were 90 per cent, 96 per cent and 97 per cent respectively, chemo might only increase your absolute chance of 10-year survival by 1 per cent.

Current recommendations are that chemotherapy should only be discussed if your benefit is 5 per cent or more, provided you are fit enough to cope with it. If your predicted benefit is less than 3 per cent, you will not be offered it as it could do more harm than good. If your benefit is between 3 per cent and 5 per cent, it is harder for your doctor to make a decision because your benefit from chemotherapy is questionable. Research has shown that lobular cancers don't respond well to chemotherapy, probably because they are slow-growing, and even if PREDICT shows a greater than 5 per cent benefit, you may still only be offered hormone treatment, which we know is highly effective in lobular cancers.

There are a couple of extra tests that your doctor can request to help them if your benefit is borderline:

Ki67

This is a protein that acts as a marker for how quickly your cancer is growing, and it's detectable on the biopsy specimen. It isn't routinely tested in the NHS, but is sometimes used as part of a research trial or to help your doctors decide whether you need chemotherapy if your benefit was borderline. A high Ki67 score (above 10 per cent) may increase your likely benefit from chemotherapy.

Cancer profiling tests

There are several tests now available that analyse your breast cancer tissue (after your surgery), such as Oncotype Dx. This looks at a set of 21 genes to predict how well your cancer will respond to chemotherapy, and the chance of your cancer returning. Patients with a borderline predicted benefit can have the Oncotype Dx test for free on the NHS. You are given a recurrence score: low, intermediate or high. A large trial called TAILORx showed that if your score is high, you should be offered chemotherapy. If it is low or intermediate, you should be able to avoid chemotherapy, although individual factors such as your age will also be taken into account. If you are not eligible for Oncotype Dx, you can ask your doctor to order the test on your behalf and pay yourself (it costs around £2,000 to £3,000).

It can be very hard to come to terms with a diagnosis of breast cancer, especially when you find out what your prognosis is. It's one thing to read about it, but how on earth do you cope with that knowledge? You may, like us, experience anger, guilt and depression that gradually fade into acceptance as your treatment progresses. Sometimes, though, feelings of anxiety and depression can be overwhelming. In the following chapter, we share how we coped.

CHAPTER 4

COPING EMOTIONALLY
WITH CANCER

WE ALL REACT differently to a cancer diagnosis. How *you* react is going to depend on many things including your personality, your personal and family circumstances, how advanced your cancer is, what treatment you need, and your own individual coping style (are you a 'glass half-full' or 'glass half-empty' person, for example?).

The first reaction when your doctor tells you that you have cancer is normally shock, and even disbelief (did they get my test results mixed up with someone else's?). Then there is often a period of distress in which you may be extremely anxious, depressed or furiously angry – and perhaps a mixture of all these. These reactions are very similar to the stages of grief (denial, anger, bargaining, depression and, finally, acceptance).

Lindsay, an American cancer nurse who got bowel cancer herself, wrote a blog, 'Here comes the sun', about her initial feelings of confusion and terror. She framed it as a letter 'to every cancer patient I ever took care of'. Here is an extract from that letter:

I'm sorry. I didn't get it.

This thought has been weighing heavy on my heart since my diagnosis. I've worked in oncology [cancer care] nearly my entire adult life ... I prided myself in connecting with my patients and helping them manage their cancer and everything that comes with it. I really thought I got it – I really thought I knew what it felt like to go through this journey. I didn't.

I didn't get what it felt like to actually hear the words ... You were trying to listen to the details and pay attention, but really you just wanted to keep a straight face for as long as it took to maybe ask one appropriate question and get the heck out of there fast. You probably went home and broke down under the weight of what you had just been told. You probably sat in silence and disbelief for hours until you had to go pretend everything was fine at work or wherever because you didn't have any details yet and wanted to keep it private still. You probably didn't even know where to start and your mind went straight to very dark places. That day was the worst. I'm sorry. I didn't get it.

I didn't get how hard the waiting is. It's literally the worst part. The diagnosis process takes forever. The different consults, the biopsies, the exams and procedures ... and the scans. Ugh, the scans. You were going through the motions trying to stay positive – but at that point, you had no idea what you were dealing with and the unknown was terrifying. Knowing the cancer is there and knowing you're not doing anything to treat it yet is an awful, helpless feeling. I'm sorry. I didn't get it.

If that's what you're feeling right now, please be reassured – things will usually get better over the next few weeks as the pieces of your own cancer jigsaw fall into place.

Trish went through a very black period for a week (she couldn't speak to anyone except her husband and he'll confirm that she wasn't her usual charming self) even though, statistically speaking, the outlook for her cancer turned out to be extremely good.

Liz felt like she was looking down watching someone else go through chemotherapy. It couldn't be real. It took her a long time to accept that she did have cancer.

In the first few days, weeks and even months, you will probably feel a deep sense of sadness and loss. Like we did, you may lie awake at night feeling thumping in your heart and desolation in your soul, planning your own funeral. You may feel guilty – that it's your fault you have cancer and your fault your loved ones have to cope with it. You may hate all the pink breast cancer products on sale in shops that seem to make light of what you are going through. All of these things can make it very difficult to concentrate and make decisions, especially while you are waiting for treatment to start. You may find you are living in a 'dream world' – just going through the motions without really feeling anything. These feelings are often even worse if you've found out that your cancer has come back.

Whatever you are feeling in the beginning, it does tend to get better in time so we suggest you acknowledge these feelings and ride them out. As time goes by, two things will probably happen. First, as you learn more about your cancer, its treatment and your prognosis, your uncertainty is replaced with a positive treatment plan (see Chapter 3). Second, you will gradually put your cancer into perspective, and fit it in to your everyday life.

If your head is (metaphorically) exploding, we strongly suggest you talk to your GP or specialist nurse, or use the Breast Cancer Care and Macmillan advisors and forums for help. Here are our tips to get you through the early days:

- Ask one or two people to be your 'cancer buddy' – that is, to help you emotionally and sometimes physically during treatment. You need to know they will be there to pick you up if you fall in a heap. If you're in a stable relationship this will probably be your partner, but you could ask one of your parents, a sibling or a close friend.
- Are you going to research your cancer? You may want to read everything you can find about breast cancer to help you feel less anxious and more in control, but it's worth bearing in mind that not everything you read will be tailored to your specific cancer, and some websites and blogs can be scary to read,

and factually wrong. See Chapter 6 for tips on how to find extra information. Alternatively, you may be happy to stick with the information your medical team gives you.

- Try writing about your cancer. Keeping a private diary or a public blog can help you gain a sense of coherence and make sense of your emotions.

Liz found it very hard to cope with her cancer diagnosis because she knew too much about what might happen in the future. She turned to blogging to help her make sense of what was happening, and this was a lifeline for her.

Trish didn't write during her treatment, but she wrote an academic paper about her cancer experience when her treatment had finished.

- Do something to take your mind off cancer. If you can't concentrate on a book, try watching old films or box sets that are familiar and comforting. Alternatively, take up jigsaws, gardening or going for a walk to get some fresh air and a sense of perspective. Doing a little exercise every day will get your endorphins going and hopefully make you feel better afterwards.
- Having cancer can be very lonely. You may not meet another patient during your treatment, and therefore have no idea whether what you are feeling is normal. If your hospital has a local cancer drop-in centre, they can be a great source of support (see Chapter 14). Neither of us had one nearby. Instead, we found support from online forums and social media. We found that linking up with other patients and sharing our experiences was a lifeline.
- Play the cancer card! The rule is, you can play it whenever you want and as often as you want. If you get invited out to dinner

and don't feel you want to go, turn the invitation down. If a friend wants to come over and talk but you just want to sleep, ask them to come another day. If you can't concentrate at work because you're waiting to hear what your results are, you may need to go off sick. Don't feel guilty – you *are* sick, even if the sickness at this stage mainly consists of an overwhelming emotional reaction. (We both played the cancer card many times, and learned not to feel guilty about it.)

- Start a 'Jar of Joy', like Liz did. Good things do happen, even when you're dealing with cancer. Every time something good happens, no matter how small or silly, whether it's hearing the birds singing in the morning, finding money down the back of the sofa or getting a hug from your children, write it on a little card and put it in a jar. In time, the jar will fill up with lovely things. When you're at your very lowest, go to the jar and read a few cards. We promise it will make you smile. The idea came from our friend Dr Kate Granger, who, before she died, taught us both a lot about living with advanced cancer.

While a strong emotional reaction to a breast cancer diagnosis is normal and healthy, most people don't need to 'medicalise' that reaction by seeing a doctor about it. However, there are at least two situations when it *is* worth seeking professional advice: overwhelming anxiety and severe depression.

WHEN ANXIETY BECOMES OVERWHELMING

One reason why breast cancer is so anxiety-provoking is that seems like it takes forever to find out that you definitely have cancer and for your treatment to actually start. You may feel like you're being passed from pillar to post if you need to have extra scans and tests. This is why your initial experience may be one of uncertainty and loss of control in the face of a life-changing (and potentially life-threatening) diagnosis. These are powerful preconditions for developing anxiety. Anxiety is also common immediately after your treatment ends when your doctor has discharged you back to the care of your GP. It is hard (subconsciously) not to feel abandoned after what may have been an intensive period of support and attention, especially if you had chemotherapy.

Anxiety as a medical diagnosis can be defined as an unpleasant subjective experience associated with the perception of threat. Our bodies and minds have inbuilt safety mechanisms for escaping from threats, called a 'fight-or-flight' response. So if you feel your heart thumping quickly in the middle of the night, it's probably because your subconscious has conjured up an 'impending doom' scenario and your body has responded with a surge of adrenaline. This tips you into a state of heightened arousal with a fast heart rate, faster breathing, muscle tremor (hold out your hands in front of you – do they shake?), sweating and rumbling in your tummy. These physical reactions are accompanied by unpleasant psychological ones that includes apprehension, feeling powerless and fear of losing control.

Low-level anxiety is a normal response to getting breast cancer, but you may need medical help if you experience any of the following symptoms:

- *Inability to focus.* Are you regularly unable to focus on normal life because of uncontrollable fears and worries? For example, do you break off mid-conversation or have to leave the room?
- *Physical symptoms*, such as a racing heart, light-headedness (which probably indicates overbreathing) and tingling in your fingers (ditto). Does your chest feel tight and/or do you have trouble taking a really deep breath?
- *Trouble sleeping.* Do you find it impossible to get a full night's sleep? In particular, are you waking most nights and then unable to get back to sleep for hours?
- *Abnormal eating.* Are you so anxious that you've stopped eating (i.e. are you losing weight?) or is your 'comfort eating' making you gain large amounts of weight?

- *Panic attacks.* Do you have intermittent attacks of feeling absolutely terrified and overwhelmed, with a thumping heart, sweating and a sense of light-headedness, which last around half an hour before slowly improving?

If you've said 'yes' to several of the above questions, you should talk to your GP. They may suggest anti-anxiety medication (which is surprisingly effective at reducing the unpleasant feelings and panic attacks), talking therapy with a counsellor or even (if you're having severe symptoms) a referral to a psychiatrist.

Cognitive behavioural therapy (CBT), usually provided by a clinical psychologist, has been shown to reduce the severity of anxiety symptoms in breast cancer. It is designed to help you change patterns of thinking and behaviour – especially ones that have become entrenched like ruminating on worst-case scenarios. Rather than delving into your past (like psychoanalysis), CBT focuses on problems and difficulties you are having in the here-and-now and looks for ways to improve your state of mind in the present.

As well as talking to your GP, you might like to try these self-help techniques:

- *Talk to someone.* Have a good moan to your partner, best friend, 'cancer buddy' or religious leader (vicar, priest, rabbi, imam, etc.). They don't have to be able to solve your problems to make you feel better; just listening to you will help.
- *Write about it.* Keeping a private journal or diary lets you keep track of your thoughts and feelings, and may help you identify triggers for your anxiety.
- *Yoga, meditation or mindfulness therapy.* These can all help you feel calm and control your breathing, and hence address one of the triggers of panic attacks (overbreathing). See Chapters 14 and 18 for more information.
- *Exercise.* Physical activity can distract you, and it also burns up nervous energy. If you're in a 'fight-or-flight' state from an adrenaline surge, use the physiological reaction in a positive way to exercise (see page 229 for exercise ideas).

● *Healthy living.* Smoking and alcohol sometimes help reduce anxiety in the short term, but try to contain the amount you take as they aren't good for you in the long term.

WHEN DEPRESSION BECOMES SEVERE

Depression is a medical condition that needs treating with either talking therapy, drugs, or both. It's normal to want to withdraw and grieve, cry and change pace when bad things happen to us. It's also normal for your loved ones to react with sadness too. But with depression, these symptoms are more severe and persistent. Depression can also come on after you've finished your main treatment phase.

To see if you might be depressed (a medical diagnosis) as opposed to feeling sad and down in the dumps (variants of normal), answer these five questions:

1. *Do you no longer enjoy things?* For example, if your best friend came to cheer you up, would you be pleased to see them, or would you want them to leave you alone?
2. *Have you had dark, negative thoughts constantly for several weeks?* We all know the initial belly-blow of the cancer diagnosis, but if you're still feeling totally flat many weeks later, this probably doesn't count as a normal response.
3. *Have you lost the will to live?* Suicidal thoughts (or indeed, just wishing that you could somehow go to sleep and never wake up) are rare if you're just feeling sad but common in true depression.
4. *Do you have severe physical symptoms?* Depression often comes with physical effects. The most common of these is a change in your sleep pattern. You may sleep for hours and hours, or suffer with insomnia. You may not have the emotional energy to move off the bed or the sofa, and spend all day in bed avoiding people.
5. *Do you cry all the time?* Do you frequently find yourself in floods of tears for no particular reason?

If you're saying yes to most or all of the above, you should talk to your GP to get professional help. As doctors, we both know that part of the problem in treating depression is that many people don't realise they need help, or don't want to ask for help. Indeed, the feeling that you're not *worth* helping is part of the illness. It's not true: you *are* worth helping. People care about you and they want to support you. Perhaps show this section of the book to a friend or relative and ask them to help you approach your GP.

Just as with anxiety, there are both medical treatments and self-help treatments for depression. Medical treatments include talking therapies (either one-to-one counselling or group therapy, oriented to helping you explore your feelings around your cancer diagnosis and how it fits with everything else that's happening in your life) and medication. Drugs can really help treat depression, although they do take several weeks to start working. If your doctor advises you to take them for a short period, you should think seriously about following their advice. Having said that, depression can get better without drugs, and some people treat it with regular exercise instead.

Depression is inherently a rather passive condition. You don't have much get-up-and-go. For this reason, playing an active part in your own treatment can be very therapeutic (though not easy). Here are some self-help techniques for depression, adapted from the website of the excellent mental health charity MIND (www.mind.org.uk):

- *Look after yourself.* Take control of your patterns of daily living and try to avoid sliding into a pattern where you have no routine or discipline. Go to bed at the same time every night. Eat a balanced, healthy diet. Make sure you wash yourself and brush your teeth every day. Wear clean clothes. Make your bed. These may seem like huge tasks at first, but they will slowly get easier in time.
- *Be kind to yourself.* Do something that makes you feel good every day, if you can. Curl up with a good book. Listen to music that makes you dance around the kitchen. Start a 'Jar

COPING EMOTIONALLY WITH CANCER

of Joy' (see page 38). MIND has a similar suggestion for a 'resilience toolkit' of written ideas for positive experiences.

- *Keep active.* Do a little exercise every day. Physical activity is a well-established treatment for depression. You could try listening to a podcast or an audiobook when you go for a walk. When you feel well enough, you could join an exercise class so you have social interaction as well as exercise (see Chapter 18). Make the effort to visit a friend. It will all feel hard because the nature of depression is to want to shut yourself away and *not* do things. However, if you can walk yourself through one activity per day, this will help you recover.

- *Challenge yourself.* Keep a diary or journal to write down your negative thoughts and identify things that send you spiralling downwards. Record the things that give you a boost. Try an online CBT programme (the website of the British Association of Behavioural and Cognitive Psychotherapists, is a good place to start – see page 278 for details).

- *Stay in touch.* If you don't feel well enough to talk to family and friends in person, text or email them to let them know you're still alive and well, because they will be concerned. You could even just send an emoji. When you can, talk about how you feel with your close friends. It's not easy but it's better than keeping it bottled up. You may want to think about joining a local or online patient support group. Hearing or reading about other people's experiences can help you to move on from your own.

Now you're starting to come to terms with having breast cancer, how do you decide who to tell and how much to tell them? These decisions can be really hard to make, and everyone does it differently. In fact, we were complete opposites. In the next chapter, we're going to help you work out what to say, who to say it to and how to help the people you tell cope with your news.

CHAPTER 5

SHARING THE NEWS

THERE IS NO right time or right way to tell someone you have breast cancer. There are no rules about who needs or deserves to know, or how soon you have to tell them. It is your decision who finds out and when. This section draws on (among other sources) a great blog called 'the small c', written by a woman who initially kept her cancer diagnosis relatively quiet while she went through treatment.

Why tell anyone at all? First and foremost because it will help you to get emotional support from people who love you and they can also take on practical tasks when you're not feeling your best. Sharing the news with others may be an important step towards going beyond 'denial' and accepting your cancer diagnosis. It is also lovely to get messages, cards and flowers from friends and family, and know that you're not going through this alone.

> Liz told her immediate family and friends on the day she was diagnosed, and then told the world via Twitter the next morning. She didn't want to hide the fact that she had cancer, and she felt it would be fairly obvious once she lost her hair. She suddenly had a large network of friends to talk to online during the lonely days spent at home during chemo.

On the other hand, you may not want to tell everyone immediately, because you are still coming to terms with the news yourself. You may not be ready to deal with questions from well-wishers, such as 'Do you need chemo?', when you don't yet know yourself how your cancer is going to be treated, and you may not want people discussing your private business among themselves. You may just want to tell a small, hand-picked 'cancer circle' (or even just one 'cancer buddy') who will be there for you through the good times and the bad, and be able to laugh with you about the embarrass-ments and ironies of cancer treatment. We hope that if you handle your cancer in a way they wouldn't have done themselves, they will keep quiet because they respect *your* choices.

Whenever you tell people you have cancer, you will undoubt-edly hear advice from people who mean well, but seem to do more harm than good. They may recommend a magic cure or diet, or tell you about their friends and relatives who have died from breast cancer. None of this is helpful. In our experience, you have to go through your own treatment journey before you are ready to hear about that of others. It's may be easier to simply say 'Thank you' and then ignore their 'helpful' advice rather than try to explain how upset you are.

Perhaps against her better judgement, Trish kept her cancer diagnosis from her two sons (aged 26 and 23 at the time) until she had had her mastectomy and finished chemotherapy. The rationale at the time was that 'the timing was bad' (one son was travelling abroad and difficult to reach; the other was about to take university exams). Looking back, the main reason for delaying telling them was probably that she didn't have enough spare emotional energy to support them as well as dealing with her own reactions. When she did tell them, they were relieved to find that the treatment had gone well and her prognosis was very good. But they told her they would have preferred to have known from the outset.

Another reason not to tell people is that you may have to support *them*, because they can't cope with the fact that you have cancer. This can often happen with parents and older relatives. As you learn more about your cancer diagnosis and come to terms with it, you may find yourself doing emotional work to reassure others that your death isn't imminent, that chemotherapy isn't that bad, and so on. It's important to keep some emotional energy to build and maintain your own comfort zone.

Our advice is to do what feels right for you at the time, which may not necessarily be what a friend or relative thinks you should do.

HOW DO YOU TELL SOMEONE YOU HAVE BREAST CANCER?

Here are some tips based on our experience and the advice we gleaned from websites when we were struggling with this challenge:

1. Decide upfront how much information you want to share, and don't be pressurised to say more.
2. Try out different approaches until you find what works for you (e.g. face-to-face or email, 'factual' or 'emotional' emphasis). The first time will be awful, but it gets easier as you tell your story more and it gains coherence in a way that makes sense to you.
3. Find an appropriate time and place to share your news. You need a time when you won't be interrupted to make phone calls and send emails, or perhaps arrange to go for a walk or meet in the park.
4. Write out what you want to say about your breast cancer (maybe one or two paragraphs), so you can copy this into emails and letters, or read it out over the phone. You might say only that you're having treatment for breast cancer and leave it there, or you might want to share all the treatment details. If you're not

telling everyone, make it clear who you are telling and what level of confidentiality you would like people to follow.

5. If people want to hear more details about your cancer and ask questions that you don't know the answer to, refer them to the Breast Cancer Care and Macmillan websites, which have excellent information leaflets and advice. It's not your job to explain all the technicalities to everyone.

6. Once you have told someone, there will usually be a silence while they let the news sink in, and they may start to cry, which can then make you cry. Telling people you love that you have cancer is a very emotional thing to do. It is even harder if you have to tell them you need chemo, and harder still if you're breaking the news that your cancer has come back. They will be upset, and you need to be prepared for this. It may be easier to tell one close friend or family member, and then ask them to tell the rest of your friends and family.

7. One of the first things people will ask is 'What can we do to help?', and you won't have a clue because you have (hopefully) never had cancer before. Try to come up with a list of things beforehand. It may be as simple as sending a daily text to say they are thinking about you. You could ask people to walk with you every day, to keep an eye on your partner while you're having treatment and take them out for a drink, or help out around the house by filling the freezer with food, doing the laundry or helping with pet care or school runs. It's also important to remind people that you are still 'you' – you are not just a cancer patient and you (perhaps) still want to be included in all the gossip, meet up for coffee and be invited to parties.

8. Think about how you want to update people on your progress. You may choose to send periodic emails, or even write a blog (there are several websites, such as Wordpress, that are free to use). A middle ground is to use a website such as CaringBridge, a private site where your blog can be seen only by the people you share it with.

HOW PEOPLE MIGHT REACT

We were lucky – most of the people we told were wonderful. After their initial reaction of shock (swearing, crying and more swearing!), they were able to support us and our husbands when we needed it. We hope that the people you tell are just as sensitive and supportive. However, not everyone is that lucky, and you may come across the following negative reactions.

Blocking you out

Some people will avoid you or withdraw completely. They may stop returning texts or phone calls, and may avoid you at work. Perhaps they just don't know what to say or worry that they will say the wrong thing and therefore end up saying nothing. Alternatively, they may find it distressing to see you sick, upset or in pain (they may have looked on you as a parent figure or mentor, and unconsciously saw you as invulnerable). They may start thinking about their own mortality and whether they might get cancer which may all be too much for them.

If you want to stay in contact with someone who has blocked you, first start by acknowledging that you feel hurt, angry or rejected. Putting your reaction aside, here are some suggestions:

- Try phoning or emailing them. Tell them it's not easy, and that you wouldn't know what to do or say if they got cancer, but you still want to see or hear from them.
- Ask them to do little things to help you (see page 47), so they can feel useful and involved without having to think too much.
- Ask them if they want you to send them some information about breast cancer treatment and survival to reassure them that you're not going to die tomorrow.
- Ask one of your other friends or relatives to talk to them and see if that helps.

Sometimes you may have to accept that this person cannot deal with your cancer diagnosis at this time in their life. This can be upsetting, especially if the person was close to you before your diagnosis. Remember, you've done nothing wrong and they are staying away for their own personal reasons, however unfathomable that may seem to you.

Gossip and chatter

A newly diagnosed cancer is a talking point – but few of us want to *be* that talking point. As 'the small c' says on her blog:

> I didn't want to be talked about. Fact is, bad news travels fast. And some people are always going to gossip. 'Hey, did you hear? Such and such has cancer.' While I wanted empathy, prayers and love, I also wanted people to believe I would be OK, not that I was going to die from my cancer. Adding to the difficulty, I also understand that some people who I care about, and who I've trusted with confidential information, might need emotional support too, and will be inclined to reach out to other people, including people who I might not want to share the information with.

Friends may need to talk about you when you're not there to help them cope with your diagnosis. You can ask them not to talk about you with people you don't know or people you haven't told, although it is impossible to stop gossip. When you do tell people, be explicit about who knows what. This is especially important if you are delaying telling children or certain relatives. It can be harder to hide a cancer diagnosis if you are having chemotherapy, or need palliative care or hospice treatment. That may be the time to send an email simply explaining what is going on, that you aren't well enough to answer questions and will provide updates in the future. Giving your friends and family a regular update via email or a blog can also help them keep a handle on reality.

Putting their foot in it

It is almost inevitable that somebody (with the best of intentions) is going to say something really crass. There really isn't much you can do to stop them, so maybe this is a time when a sense of humour is called for. The following statements are examples of things people might say to you. Have a laugh about them, and brace yourself for the time when someone says something even worse to you!

'Live in the moment.' / 'Be strong.' / 'Fight hard.' / 'Keep your chin up.' / 'Don't give up.' / 'Think positive.'

'It could be worse, you know.'

'Everything happens for a reason.'

'At least it's not on your face where everyone could see the scars, besides you don't really need your breasts anyway.'

'Gosh, I thought chemo was supposed to make you lose weight.'

'My uncle/cousin/friend's mother had cancer and they died.'

'Smile – you're getting a free boob-job!'

Enough said. Just keep a tight hold of that sense of humour!

WHEN YOUR LOVED ONE GETS BREAST CANCER

While we were writing this book, Trish received the following email, out of the blue, from someone who had been following her on Twitter. We reproduce it with his consent.

My mother was recently diagnosed with breast cancer, which has spread quite far. We're hopeful, but cautious at the same time. Why

I'm contacting you, though, is because I just don't know what I can do for her, how I should act around her, what I should talk about with her when I visit her in hospital. I live in [town A] and she is in [town B, 200 miles away], so I'm up there every second week or so to see her. I guess my question is: how did you want people to treat you? I know this is such a highly personal thing, and every person with cancer will differ. I've been trying to carry on as 'normal', and pretending like it's just another visit, filling her in on details on my life and my friends, the things we would talk on the phone about. I don't want to skirt around the issue, but I don't want her cancer to be THE issue.

There are no rules when it comes to how to act towards a family member, or indeed any close friend with cancer. Like the writer of the above email realised, every cancer patient is different. People need or want support in many different ways, and if two people you know got cancer, they may each cope in very different ways. How on earth are you meant to know what to do? This wasn't covered in school.

We replied with the lessons we've learned from experience, and our tips are summarised below.

As the writer did, accept that there will be an awkward tension between behaving 'normally' and dealing with the elephant in the room, their cancer. Most people 'muddle through' using a combination of intuition, common sense and basic humanity.

Even though you may live with them, send them daily texts and regular cards to brighten up their day. There's nothing nicer than getting a 'just thinking of you' card in the post instead of a bill.

Ask your relative if there are things you can do to help – from sorting out a will to taking charge of the food shopping, from helping set up a blog or giving them a hug. They will know what they want and need from you.

It's okay to laugh and joke about what is happening. You *have* to have a sense of humour. Cancer can be pretty black at times, and laughing about it helps everyone.

Your relative may not be interested in the finer points of their treatment and prognosis and want to leave everything to the doctors, whereas you may want to know every little detail. Try to respect their wishes, and not interfere with how they are handling things. Their doctor cannot talk to you about their treatment without their consent. If you are feeling angry or impatient with one aspect of their treatment, try not to show it.

Remember that your relative is not just a cancer patient. It's important to talk to them about everything you used to. It's incredibly tiring when the only thing anyone wants to talk to you about is your cancer. One way to handle this is to say to them 'I'm not going to bring up your cancer unless you mention it, and then I'll know you're ready to talk about it.'

At some point, they may want to talk about the 'elephant in the room' – the fact that they might die because of their breast cancer. Most people who are diagnosed with cancer imagine their death and their funeral, and it's important to acknowledge this if your relative wants to bring it up.

Don't tell your relative to 'cheer up'. Unless you've had cancer you can never really know what it's like to deal with the emotional strain on you and your family. If they're sad, just listen to what they have to say without passing judgement or trying to 'solve' their problems.

Don't ask too many questions. They may be sick of constantly repeating their story, or they may want to keep some details private. Being a family member does not automatically entitle you to know everything that is going on.

Finally, don't compare your relative with the person they were before cancer. Cancer treatment can at times be uniquely exhausting and disheartening, depending on the treatment they need. We were very fit, and we tolerated chemotherapy well, but we both had days when we literally couldn't get out of bed. Fortunately, no one said to us 'pull yourself together' on those darkest days.

TELLING YOUR CHILDREN

Deciding whether to tell your children that you have breast cancer is not easy, especially if they are young. Deciding *how* to tell them can be even harder, since you will need to pitch the message at an appropriate level for your child's age and maturity. There's no right way to do this. Remember that *you* are an expert in your own children and in the way you communicate that works for you as a family. That personal knowledge is at least as important as what we have written here. You may not want to tell your children at all. However, children can be remarkably perceptive and will almost certainly pick up that something is different.

There are many excellent books written by cancer charities and several mums who have had breast cancer that can help you. Your breast care nurse will be able to recommend some to you. We came across an excellent free online resource called 'Talking to Kids about Cancer' produced by a public health group in Victoria, Australia, which you can download for free: www.cancervic.org.au/downloads/resources/booklets/talking-to-kids-about-cancer/Talking-to-Kids-About-Cancer.pdf

Adult children

Use the same principles covered earlier in the chapter about telling friends and family. You may want to do this face-to-face instead of over the phone if possible.

Teenagers and older children

Teenagers and older children are likely to pick up that something is wrong and may worry more than if they knew the truth. If you don't tell them and they find out by accident from a friend's parent or a teacher, they may feel betrayed and have difficulty hiding the fact that they know what is going on. It may also be hard if you have younger children as well, and you tell your teenagers but ask them not to tell their younger siblings. On the whole, it is probably better to share your cancer news with your older children sooner rather than later. That way you can support them, answer their questions and help them cope as you go through treatment.

You could try doing a 'dress rehearsal' with your partner, but you can't predict how your children will react, and if you have several children, each may react differently. Again, you could try writing down what you want to tell them, as well as a list of things you *don't* want them to know, so that it can be clear in your head when you come to break the news.

Your breast care nurse may be able to give you a leaflet or a book that you can give to them, and you can point them to safe websites, such as Breast Cancer Care and Macmillan, so they can satisfy their own curiosity. This is safer than a random Internet search in the middle of the night, although it's worth acknowledging that they may do this as well. Answer their questions honestly, even if the answer is 'I don't know'. Be honest about your own feelings, and give your children a chance to tell you how *they* are feeling. When you are feeling weak, tired, nauseous, miserable, antisocial, angry and so on, remind your children that your physical state and/or mood is not because of something they have done (or failed to do).

There is a great book written for teenagers called *Eek! My Mummy Has Breast Cancer* written by Emma Sutherland, who was 12 when her mum was diagnosed.

It is probably sensible to let someone at their school know. The senior leadership team may have an opinion about which teacher(s) should be told, and whether to share the news with your children's friends or not. You can pass on the leaflets that your breast care nurse gave you to your children's teachers and/or friends. If you think your children are struggling, professional counselling might help, which your GP could arrange. Older children can also speak to their GP about how they are feeling in strict confidence and you will not be entitled to know what has been discussed.

Younger children

Young children and toddlers will not understand much of what is going on, so you need to keep things simple. You could start by saying 'Mummy is poorly' every day until you think they understand. It can be hard to answer their questions in language that they can understand, and it may be worth working out how you are going to describe surgery, radiotherapy or chemo-therapy first, and getting close friends and family on board with the same child-friendly terms. Your children may want to act out some scenarios or draw pictures rather than talk around a table. Ask them (for example) to do a drawing of mummy and talk about it, or everyone could play going to the cancer clinic.

However you tell them, your children are likely to find the news upsetting and unsettling. Keep reminding them that you love them, and that this is not their fault (young children sometimes worry that it is their fault for being naughty). Spend as much time with them as you can, even if it's just watching TV. Reassure them that someone will always be there to look after them. This may be obvious to the adults involved, but may need spelling out to young children.

We recommend Gillian Forrest's charming story book for young children, *Mummy's Lump*, which is available as a free download from Breast Cancer Care: www.breastcancercare.org.uk/sites/default/files/publications/pdf/mummys_lump_2015_web.pdf

Dealing with the disruption of family life

Children are creatures of habit, and they don't like it when their routine is disturbed. If you just need surgery and radiotherapy, then the disruption will be minimal, probably just for a couple of weeks while you recover from your operation. If you need chemotherapy, there will be a big upheaval. Holidays and birth-day parties may need to be cancelled, sleepovers at home are no longer allowed because of the infection risk, although the kids may enjoy choosing and eating takeaways if you are too poorly to cook. They may feel like a lost parcel as different friends and neighbours chip in to help with school runs. Make sure that everyone helping you knows what your children have been told, to avoid confusion.

Explain that these changes are temporary (unless you have secondary cancer when there may be a permanent change at home), and that you will plan fun things for when your treatment has ended. Allow room for negotiation if you can (that 'inessential' weekly activity may be your child's necessary escape from a traumatic situation). Ask friends whether they could give your child regular quality time (or commit to getting them to that inconvenient activity once a week). Talk to your children about what *they* did while you were away having treatment. Get them to take photos and videos so they can share parts of their experience with you. Reassure them it's still okay to have fun and enjoy themselves while you are feeling ill.

If you are feeling rotten, you may not pick up signs that your child is not coping. Ask your child's teacher and their friends' parents to let you know if they have any concerns. They may have mood swings, and alternately feel guilty, confused, angry, sad or just unable to express what they feel. They may also 'regress' and start to behave as a much younger child (or even a baby). If you are finding it hard to watch your children struggling to cope, you can often get support from online forums and from Breast Cancer Care's 'Someone Like Me', who can put you in touch with other mums.

WORK

In the UK, after a cancer diagnosis you are legally protected from unfair treatment at work. As long as your employer knows you have had cancer, they have to support you through your treatment and are not allowed to discriminate against you, although the amount of sick leave you are entitled to will depend on your contract of employment. The people you tell at work are also required by law to keep your personal information confidential from your other work colleagues. The Macmillan website gives more detail on this (see page 280).

Telling your employer

It is up to you whether you tell your employer about your cancer. If you are only away from work for a couple of weeks, no one may realise that you have had cancer and you may want to keep it that way. Your employer may still need to know that you have been unwell or need to attend further appointments or have additional tests. It may help to tell them in advance how often these appointments are likely to be, even if you don't say what they are for.

It will be harder to disguise several months away for chemotherapy, so we advise you to be up front with your employer about this. When you are first diagnosed, returning to work may be the last thing on your mind, but you should anticipate that you will be tired and need a phased return with reduced hours and/or a lighter workload for at least the first couple of weeks. If you feel you can talk to your employer in advance, tell them that you will keep in touch and start planning your return to work when you're ready.

Your legal protection does not take away the emotional and practical awkwardness of discussing cancer with your employer. Macmillan has produced an excellent guide, called 'Finding the words', to help you with this challenge. Make notes of any meetings you have, and copy them to your manager so you both have a record of what was said. Remember if you are not feeling well, you can cancel your meeting and rearrange it for another time.

You should also read your employment contract again and check your company's sickness policy. Find out how much sick leave you are entitled to and whether this is full-pay or half-pay. This can help you plan your return to work, especially if money worries are an issue. If you are a member of a union, you can ask them for advice.

Telling work colleagues

It can be difficult to break the news of your cancer diagnosis to work colleagues. You may worry that everyone will give you pitying looks in the office, gossip about you behind your back or treat you differently. You may be the first person some of your colleagues have ever known with cancer, and they may not know what to do. If you do decide to tell people, we recommend planning in advance what you want to say, how much information you want to tell people and what you are happy to talk about. Setting some simple ground rules can make things a little easier. For example, you may want to ask someone to send an email round to key staff with these details to save you from repeating yourself.

Working through breast cancer

If you don't need chemotherapy, you should only need to take a couple of weeks off work to recover from your operation, and it is possible to carry on working around radiotherapy treatment. If you have chemotherapy, you may choose not to work. However, some people carry on working on a part-time basis, and plan work around their good and bad days or weeks. Working through chemo can give you a sense of normality, social company and a sense of purpose. You may also need to work for financial reasons (e.g. if you're not eligible for much sick leave or you're self-employed). If you decide to keep working, you will need to let your line manager know realistically how much you are capable of doing.

Returning to work after breast cancer

There are lots of things that may affect your return to work, such as fatigue, depression and menopausal symptoms. Essentially, you may find it difficult to concentrate and take longer to do things than you did before. You may also find you are exhausted after a full day back at work, and need a lighter day to recover. (We cover the side effects of treatments on pages 141–6.)

Because of side effects and the time you've had away, you will probably be less efficient – and less confident – than before you went off sick. Your employer is legally obliged to make 'reasonable adjustments' to help you get back to work, including what is known

IF YOU'RE FINANCIALLY STRETCHED
AND/OR SELF-EMPLOYED

Not everyone is lucky enough to be covered by generous sickness benefit schemes. Financial worries on top of cancer are no fun. If your income is reduced or stops, you may feel unable to pay the bills and support your family. This can lead to a loss of self-confidence at a time when your self-image is already low. You may have to adjust the family budget to accommodate a fall in income.

If you run your own business you may feel under severe stress because your employees and/or family members are dependent on the business turnover continuing as normal. You may have put your heart and soul into building up your business and fear that your life's work is in danger of collapsing. If you are self-employed and have no one else to rely on, it can be just as hard to deal with.

Again, the Macmillan website has a lot of advice including support for small businesses and the self-employed. The government, business organisations and voluntary groups offer a range of services, many of which are free. Macmillan can also help you work out if you are entitled to benefits to help tide you over.

as a 'phased return' (e.g. perhaps going back three days a week initially, then increasing to four and then five days when you are ready), flexible start or finish times, changing your job description to remove tasks you are no longer able to do, moving you to a post with more suitable duties (if you agree), additional breaks for resting, and changing performance targets to take account of time you have missed. If you have developed a disability (such as heart failure), you may need additional measures (such as an accessible parking space).

Talk to your employer in advance so they can help you plan all this. It may take more than one meeting (or a series of phone calls, or someone coming to visit you at home or on neutral ground) to work out what you are now capable of doing in your job and what needs to be done to smooth your return.

If you're about to have what you anticipate could be a difficult conversation with your line manager, do your research, know your rights, make a plan for what you would like to happen and write down what you'd like to cover in your meeting. You may not get everything you wish for, but at least you will have made your case clearly and reasonably.

If you and your employer put a bit of planning into your return to work, you will probably find it a positive experience. Your colleagues will be pleased to see you, and there may even be a welcome celebration! The week before you return, you could ask your line manager to send an email round to staff saying you'll be coming back soon and are keen to get back into your usual routines. They might explain to colleagues that you'll be working short days (or whatever adjustments you've agreed) for a few weeks.

Additional information and support

The Macmillan website has lots of advice on returning to work after cancer, and you can call one of their advisors to get extra help. If your organisation has an Occupational Health Department, you should make an appointment to see them. Everything you tell them is confidential, and they may be able to help if you are finding it hard to cope at work.

There are other organisations such as Working With Cancer (see page 282) whose goal is to help people get back to work after any kind of cancer. They tend to work mostly with employers (for example, your employer might refer you to them for a programme of coaching), but you can self-refer for coaching to help you work through potential problems.

Trish stopped working as a GP as soon as she was diagnosed, but continued working as an academic (writing papers and books) throughout her chemotherapy and surgery, mostly at home. Her employer was very supportive and excused her from teaching duties and committee meetings while she was having chemo. Trish returned to work within two weeks of finishing chemo, but was very tired for three months so left work at around 4pm to go home and have a nap before getting up for supper. The Occupational Health Department at her university were very helpful. It was two years before she was back to her usual 12-hour academic days including lunchtime meetings and evening teaching!

Liz stopped working as a breast surgeon when she was diagnosed. She went back to work on a part-time basis one year after finishing treatment. It was a little more complicated for Liz because she had to cope with the physical and mental stress of being a surgeon, as well as the emotional stress of looking after breast cancer patients again. She still gets tired after a full day's work.

Sharing the news that you've got cancer can be quite hard work, and you will inevitably encounter some unhelpful reactions from a minority of people. However, there's more than a grain of truth in the maxim that 'a problem shared is a problem halved'. Both at home and at work, once people know what you're going through, friends, family and colleagues will generally come on side and try to help.

Now that you've shared the news, and the crying and the swearing have stopped, the next question you're likely to be asked is, 'What treatment are you going to have?'. At this stage, you may not know. All too often, people tell you about diets and supplements they've heard can cure cancer, or talk about the dangers of standard breast cancer treatments. In the next chapter, we're going to explain why breast cancer is treated the way it is, and help you understand and interpret these so-called miracle cures so you can make up your own mind.

CHAPTER 6

THE SCIENCE OF BREAST CANCER TREATMENT

YEARS AGO, THERE was no standard guidance for the treatment of breast cancer. Since the early nineties, however, doctors have based their treatment recommendations on scientific evidence from research studies that have looked at the outcomes of hundreds of thousands of women with breast cancer taking different treatments, often over a 10- to 20-year period. These studies are usually randomised controlled trials (RCTs) in which cancer patients are randomly allocated (e.g. using a random number generator on a computer) to an intervention group (who receive a new treatment) or a control group (who receive the standard treatment, or no treatment at all). All of this is done in a carefully controlled setting and the results are accurately recorded. Randomisation is important, since non-random allocation (e.g. giving the new treatment to people with more advanced cancer) would mean you couldn't prove anything reliable about the benefits of the treatment.

Breast cancer is now one of the most researched conditions in any branch of medicine. Hundreds of RCTs have been done looking at many different treatment options. To help doctors make their decisions, they look at the combined results from lots of RCTs using a statistical technique called meta-analysis, which can increase the confidence with which they can say that treatment A is better than treatment B.

The results of breast cancer RCTs and meta-analyses are used by leading experts to write national and international guidelines advising doctors how to treat patients with primary and secondary breast cancer. In the UK, evidence-based guidelines produced by the National Institute for Health and Care Excellence (NICE) summarise all the relevant high-quality evidence. Every doctor treating you should follow these guidelines (whether on the NHS or privately), although it's important to bear in mind that these are only guidelines and every patient is considered on an individual basis. In America, the guidelines are produced by the American Society of Clinical Oncology (ASCO). We have drawn mainly on NICE guidelines when writing this book.

We have not listed all the major research trials and meta-analyses because there are so many of them, but they can all be found in the relevant NICE guidelines which are free to download. Where we do mention a trial, you should be able to find it by searching online for key words (e.g. the author's name, the drug or other intervention, and 'breast cancer').

UNDERSTANDING RESEARCH TRIALS

Most cancer research trials are designed to measure whether a certain treatment gives patients a better outcome. There are different ways of describing this, and they are often recorded as a percentage. 'Overall survival' means how many people are alive at the end of the trial. 'Disease-free survival' means how many patients are alive and haven't developed a recurrence. 'Quality of life' measures give an indication of whether the side effects of treatments are so bad that they outweigh any survival benefits.

Careful consideration is needed when a trial (or a story in the press) claims that it improves these outcomes. Results can be expressed in absolute terms or relative terms (absolute is better). A trial could claim that 'eating X doubles your risk' of getting breast cancer. This sounds scary! However, it is a relative benefit. The actual, absolute benefit is that 'eating X increases your risk of getting breast cancer from 1 in 1,000 to 2 in 1,000'. Both statements are true, but the absolute benefit is less misleading – even if you eat X, you still have 998 chances in 1,000 of *not* getting breast cancer!

Cancer trials take a long time to get results, especially if they set out to study long-term survival over many years. A 10-year study of people who developed breast cancer in 2006, for example, is unlikely to be published until 2020. Since treatments are improving all the time, this means that your chances of survival are *at least* as good as the odds reported in published trials – and very often considerably better, because new treatments are always being developed.

NICE guidelines mean that if a patient is seen by any breast surgeon, anywhere in the UK, they should be offered the same treatment plan. However, every case is discussed by a team of doctors in a multidisciplinary team (see page 17), before the plan is then discussed with you, the patient. You can then ask about alternative options, and fit the treatment plan around your own priorities and lifestyle choices. Your doctor can help you weigh up the balance between potential *benefits*, the potential *risks* or side effects, and what might be called the 'hassle value' (how many visits to hospital, how many blood tests, how much time needed off work, and so on). Sometimes there may be two equally effective treatment options, and the decision will be yours to make.

You may not want to get involved in this decision-making process, preferring to simply go ahead with whatever your doctor recommends, based on the evidence and guidelines. Your doctor should talk to you about the pros and cons of surgery, chemotherapy and radiotherapy as part of the consent process. If you do want to get more involved with 'shared decision-making', here are five key questions to consider asking about *any* test or treatment:

1. What are my options?
2. What are the absolute benefits of each option?
3. What are the absolute risks (side effects) of each option?

4. What is the evidence for this treatment?
5. What happens if I don't have the test or treatment?

'MIRACLE' AND ALTERNATIVE CURES

We understand that having cancer can be scary as it is a serious and potentially fatal condition. You may feel a strong temptation to 'clutch at straws' and sign up to anything that promises a cure (common ones are extreme diets, mega-vitamins, homeopathy and spiritual therapies), maybe as an attempt at regaining control over your body and your life, and we discuss these so-called miracle cures in more detail in Chapter 18. While we understand this pressure, we want to warn you of the dangers of taking treatments that are not evidence-based. If you do decide to take such treatments, please consider taking them alongside traditional medical treatments. We know that breast cancer can still come back despite everything medicine has to offer, but if you don't follow the advice of your medical team, the risk of recurrence could be far, far higher.

This excerpt is from a blog published in the *Huffington Post* (17 April 2017) from Dr Lawence Saez (a cancer survivor himself) entitled 'Cancer and the Snake Oil Industry':

Vitamin B17, frankincense, apricot seeds, blue scorpion tail extract, moringa, turmeric, essiac tea. These are among the hundreds of alleged cancer-killing cures that will be unfamiliar to most people, but not for those of us who are cancer patients. Information about these products typically emerges from online discussion boards or closed Facebook chatrooms. Sometimes concerned friends inundate you with information about such miracle cancer cures. For cancer patients, who are overwhelmed with the traditional treatments for cancer, these alternative cures can offer a sign of hope. However appealing, we must be aware about the dangerous implications of natural cancer cures.

Every cancer patient is likely to have come across a number of videos relating to non-traditional medicine cancer cures. The general premise of these videos is that oncologists are puppets of the pharmaceutical industry. According to this narrative, traditional medicine cancer treatments are, at best, ineffective or, in the worst of cases, they actually cause the spread of cancer.

Oftentimes, a natural health cure 'doctor' will claim that everything that a cancer patient has been told about cancer by their oncologist is wrong. These 'doctors' will then offer some sort of miraculous cancer cure, typically a juice cocktail or some vitamin protocol. These snake oil salesmen offer no concrete scientific evidence for their extraordinary claims. Normally, the only evidence offered by these 'doctors' are testimonials, allegedly from cancer patients who claim to have been cured by these non-traditional treatments. Individually, these 'cures' are unlikely to harm a cancer patient. The real damage comes when these snake oil doctors then encourage cancer patients to forego traditional medicine treatment for these purported cures.

This is wise advice. We have both seen friends and patients refuse scientifically-proven, free (in the UK) medical treatments and instead use 'alternative cures' at great expense. Some of these 'cures' cost hundreds of thousands of pounds, and involve flying monthly to countries like Mexico and Japan.

A major study published in 2018 in the *Journal of the National Cancer Institute* by a team led by Dr Skyler Johnson showed that *women with breast cancer were more than five times as likely to die if they took alternative medicines only*, compared with women who had traditional breast cancer treatment. Dr Johnson has an excellent blog where he introduces what he calls the 'Cancer Claims CRAP Test', which he has kindly given us permission to reproduce on the next page. In short, if a cancer claim is a) too good to be true, b) made by someone who is after your money, c) based on nothing more than anecdote, and d) hard to verify in the published literature, it fails the CRAP test and you should be very cautious about it.

Evaluating Cancer Claims: Are they CRAP?

Use the questions below to help you evaluate cancer claims from people, websites, social media or videos. Place a 1 next to each section if you answer yes. Add up the final score to decide whether the cancer claim is crap.

C

Conspiracies or Claims too good to be true

- Does the person or website elicit conspiracies of ineffective cancer treatments, cancer cure suppression, or natural cures?
- Are the claims made too good to be true like 'no side-effects' and 'Miracle Cure?'

R

Requests for money

- Are products for sale like herbal/botanical supplements, vitamins/minerals, consultations, books or DVDs?

A

Anecdotes

- Are the stories unverifiable in another reputable source?
- Is the information unsupported by the medical literature?

P

Publisher

- Are the author's medical credentials hidden and difficult to verify? If so, is the source anything other than a .ac.uk, .gov.uk or Oncology hospital website?

Total Score

Scoring:

0: Acceptable claim but stay vigilant
1: Be careful, possible crap
2: Crap
3: So much crap
4: Crappiest crap ever

Here are some rules of thumb for interpreting scientific claims that are pitched at the general public, instead of doctors and scientists. They may be particularly useful when assessing alternative therapies.

Science or not?

Real scientists do not set up a research study in order to confirm a preconceived idea. They do it to *test a hypothesis* from the neutral position which assumes that the results could go either one way or the other. An honest scientist is cautious and critical of their own work and that of others and will always underplay rather than overplay the significance of their work.

Animal or human?

Just because something cures cancer in mice doesn't mean it's going to cure the same cancer in humans. Arguably animal studies have a place in science (we acknowledge those who disagree with this) but even when the findings of such studies are promising, they are still *preliminary*. To draw conclusions about humans, they have to be repeated, and the results reproduced, in human trials.

Healthy volunteers or real patients?

Cancer treatments have to be tested, and shown to work, on cancer patients. Drugs are often given to healthy volunteers first, to make sure that the side effects are not too terrible, but this doesn't mean that the drug is going to work effectively against your cancer.

Big or small?

It is not necessarily true that a big study is better than a small one. But, all others things being equal, the larger the study, the more likely it is to approximate to the truth. Most large breast cancer trials recruit thousands of patients, whereas some 'alternative cures' are marketed on the basis of tiny studies looking only at a handful of patients. Before they change their clinical practice, doctors want to know that the results can be reproduced in lots and lots of patients, to make sure that the small trial isn't a one-off. A meta-analysis (see page 63) can be done to combine the findings from several smaller studies to give a clearer picture of how effective (or not) the drug is.

Association or causation?

One commonly used scientific approach in the study of cancer causation is to measure a lot of different things (known as 'variables') in a large number of people and then follow these people over a few years to see who gets cancer. This is known as a 'cohort study'. Variables typically measured include smoking status, alcohol intake, different aspects of diet, exercise levels, and so on. But the best such a study can ever produce is an estimate of *association* (meaning: two things occurring together); it can almost never prove *causation* (that one of the variables actually *caused* the cancer).

Very rarely, a really good cohort study *can* demonstrate causation. For example, the original research linking smoking and lung cancer was done using a cohort study. In that study, the association was very strong (over 90 per cent of the lung cancers occurred in the smokers); there was a 'dose response' effect (the more you smoked, the more likely you were to get lung cancer); and as people were followed up for several decades, it became clear that *giving up* smoking was (after a few years) associated with a reduction in the risk of lung cancer. All these things helped to show that in this case, the association between smoking and lung cancer *was* causal. But *most* associations – for example between drinking coffee and getting cancer, or taking a particular vitamin and preventing cancer – are much, much weaker overall; the dose-response effect is weak or non-existent; and change in behaviour has not been shown to change risk. Whatever you may read in the press, the biggest risks for getting breast cancer are still being a woman and getting older, neither of which you can change.

RCT or not?

We talked about RCTs (or randomised control trials) earlier (page 63). When evaluating cancer treatments, you should generally ignore any claim that is not based on a RCT. If the person claiming that their miracle treatment cures cancer can't back it up with at least one RCT, think twice before signing up for it.

Surrogate or definitive endpoints?

Apologies for the jargon in this title, but these terms are important. Clinical trials have definitive endpoints that can be accurately measured – such as overall survival and disease-free survival (see page 64). If a treatment is scientifically proven to improve cancer survival, your doctors will recommend it to you. A surrogate endpoint is something that's usually easy to measure (for example, your cancer appears to shrink on a scan) but which isn't always a true indicator of whether a treatment is working, i.e. whether you will live longer because of your treatment. If the *only* evidence in favour of a particular treatment is a change in a surrogate endpoint, this is relatively weak evidence.

If you'd like to get more deeply into how to assess scientific papers, Trish has written a book called *How to Read a Paper: the Basics of Evidence-based Medicine* (Wiley-Blackwell, 2014). Liz actually used this book herself when she sat her surgical exams.

TAKING PART IN RESEARCH

We both know how important scientific research is when it comes to improving survival from breast cancer, because we've done research ourselves and because the treatments we received as patients were based on research trials. One goal of the UK Association of Breast Surgery is that every patient should be offered the opportunity to be involved in a research trial.

Most breast units in the UK will be running several different research trials at any one time. Your doctor will talk to you about any suitable trials and ask you if you would like some more information. This information is normally given to you by a specialist research nurse. If you're not keen, say so. You don't have to be part of a trial and your clinical care will not be compromised if you say no (you will simply be treated according to the current standard guidelines, as discussed above).

Taking part in a research study means you are contributing to the development of new treatments for breast cancer, and hopefully, one day, a cure. Even if you don't gain personally, future generations of patients will. There are different kinds of trials, which include:

- new ways of analysing breast cancer and genetic testing
- surgical operations, chemotherapy and radiotherapy regimens
- the effects of a particular treatment on your quality of life
- the effects of counselling, diet, and exercise on your survival from breast cancer

There are some downsides to agreeing to take part in a research trial. It may be too much information to take in when you are still coping with a cancer diagnosis and the trial could mean extra hospital visits, blood tests or scans. You may also be allocated to the standard treatment and not get the new trial drug, but you won't know until the trial has finished. Trials of drug treatments can go on for several years or more, so it can be a long-term commitment.

On the upside, being part of a research study means that you will be very carefully monitored and followed up, usually with more frequent appointments than someone who is not in a trial.

Where can I find out what trials are available?

Most hospitals in the UK are involved in several breast cancer trials at any time. Your doctor should tell you about all the trials in your hospital that are suitable for you. If you have heard of a different trial, either online or from other patients, you can ask your doctor about this. You may have to be treated in a different hospital, which could be far away from you, if you want to take part. There are relatively few trials for patients with secondary breast cancer, and most of these are run at the larger cancer centres, which may mean travelling to take part. The Cancer Research UK website has a list of all the current breast cancer trials: www.cancer-researchuk.org/about-cancer/find-a-clinical-trial

QUESTIONS TO ASK YOUR DOCTOR ABOUT RESEARCH TRIALS

If you're unsure whether you want to be involved in a particular trial or not, ask your doctor or the research nurse these questions adapted from the Breast Cancer Care website:

- What does the trial involve?
- Will I know if I'm getting the new treatment or not?
- How long will I be in it for?
- Can I change my mind during the trial?
- Will I need to have extra blood tests or scans? How often?
- Will I need to have extra hospital visits? If so, will the trial pay for the extra travel?
- What will you do with the data collected about me?
- Who can I contact if the research nurse is not available?
- Will there be a questionnaire or diary to fill in?
- What are the side effects of the treatment?
- What treatment will I get if I don't enter the trial?
- Will I get to know the results?
- Will I be treated at the same hospital or will I have to attend a different unit?

If you want more information on what a clinical research trial is and what goes on in them, try the Clinical Trials Explained website: http://clinicaltrialsexplained.com

Now that we've talked about the science of breast cancer treatment and the rigorous research involved, we hope you have a better understanding of why your doctor recommends certain treatments to you. We also hope you're feeling a little more confident in assessing the pros and cons of alternative cancer treatments. Let's now go through, in detail, what each breast cancer treatment involves, and give you our tips and tricks to cope with each in turn.

CHAPTER 7

BREAST AND ARMPIT SURGERY

THE MOST EFFECTIVE treatment for breast cancer is an operation to remove it. There are two types of breast operation. Your surgeon will either remove the cancer and leave the rest of your breast tissue behind – called a 'lumpectomy' or 'wide local excision'. The remaining breast tissue is then treated with radiotherapy. The other option is to remove all of your breast, including the cancer. This is called a 'mastectomy'. If you need to have a mastectomy, your surgeon should discuss breast reconstruction with you, which is discussed in more detail in the next chapter.

Your surgeon may also need to remove some or all of the lymph nodes in your armpit. The first lymph node that your breast cancer spreads to is called the sentinel node (see page 9). Your surgeon may remove just the sentinel node or do a more extensive operation called an 'axillary node clearance'. We explain the difference between these below.

Which operation do you need?

If you have DCIS (non-invasive cancer), you don't need to have any lymph nodes removed because your cancer by definition cannot spread. Most women with DCIS have only a small area of it, which can be treated with a lumpectomy. If you have a large area of DCIS and need a mastectomy, there is a chance that you might have a small invasive cancer area in the middle of the DCIS. If this happens, there is also a chance that your lymph nodes could contain cancer cells, and so your surgeon will do a sentinel lymph node biopsy at the same time as your mastectomy.

If you have invasive cancer, you will have either a lumpectomy or a mastectomy, as well as lymph node surgery.

If your cancer has grown through the breast into the skin (called a 'fungating' cancer), it can cause ulcers that bleed and smell. Your surgeon will do an operation called a 'toilet' mastectomy to remove the cancer and the affected skin. If you're not well enough to have this operation, your doctors can try radiotherapy to treat it.

If you have breast cancer in your lymph glands but your doctors can't find a cancer in your breast (an occult cancer), you will have an axillary node clearance, and either a mastectomy or whole breast radiotherapy.

If you have secondary cancer from the beginning, there is no urgent need to remove your breast cancer because it has already spread. You will probably start with a combination of chemotherapy, radiotherapy or hormonal therapy. Your team will monitor your breast cancer and lymph nodes during treatment, and talk to you about the pros, cons and timing of breast surgery.

What happens if your surgeon can't feel your cancer?

If your cancer was detected through breast screening, there may be no lump to feel. If your cancer doesn't have well-defined edges, it can be hard for your surgeon to know exactly where it is. There are several methods that your surgeon can use to help find your cancer.

A radiologist will first put a small gel clip into the cancer (see page 77). Before your operation, a very fine guidewire is inserted into your cancer, next to the clip, using a local anaesthetic and either ultrasound or mammogram guidance. You will then have another mammogram to make sure that the wire is in the correct position. Your surgeon removes the tissue around the tip of the wire and then takes an X-ray to make sure that they've removed all the right area. There are alternatives to the wire, such as a radio-isotope (see page 91–2) and microscopic magnetic beads, and your surgeon will explain which technique they will use.

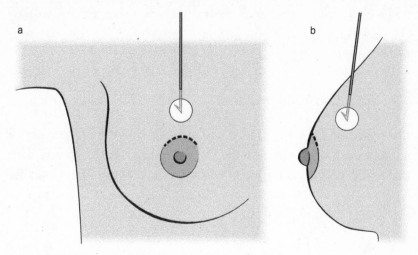

Wire-guided breast surgery

Margins

To make sure there are no cancer cells left behind, your surgeon will remove a rim of normal breast tissue, called a 'margin', around the cancer. When your cancer is analysed, the pathologist checks to make sure that the margin under the microscope is a minimum distance of 1–2mm between the cancer and the free edge – a 'clear margin'. If there are cancer cells closer than 1–2mm from the free edge, you have a 'positive margin'. The margin needs

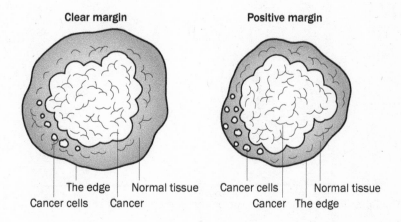

to be clear for further treatments, such as radiotherapy, to have the most benefit, so if you have a positive margin, you may need to have further surgery.

Oncoplastic breast surgery

Over the last 10 to 15 years, breast surgeons have developed plastic surgery techniques to reshape, reduce and recreate breasts after cancer surgery to improve how your breast looks. This is called

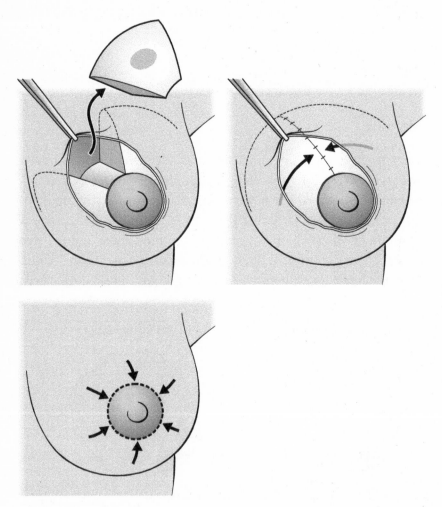

The Roundblock procedure – an example of an oncoplastic operation

'oncoplastic surgery' and is now taught to all new trainee breast surgeons. Breast surgeons can now hide your scar by placing it around your nipple or on the edge of the breast, making it hard to tell that you have had an operation. These techniques also mean that many women no longer need to have a mastectomy. For example, if you are small-breasted with a large cancer, your surgeon might be able to use some of your own fat or muscle to fill the gap left by the cancer. If you have very large breasts and a large cancer, your surgeon could offer you a breast reduction instead of a mastectomy.

The cosmetic outcome of each operation depends on the quality of your breast tissue and your skin. Your breast tissue needs to be firm enough, and your skin needs to be healthy enough, for your surgeon to use these new techniques. Ageing and smoking can affect both, and your surgeon will be honest with you about what is and isn't possible. Most but not all consultant breast surgeons are now trained in oncoplastic surgical techniques.

DECIDING WHICH OPERATION TO HAVE

This should be a joint decision between you and your surgeon. It's made in two stages. First, the multidisciplinary team (MDT, see page 17) will review all of your results and make a decision regarding breast and axillary node surgery based on the size of your breasts and the size of your cancer. As a rule of thumb, a surgeon can remove a fifth of your breast and reshape it to give you a good cosmetic result. If they need to remove more than a fifth of your breast to safely remove the cancer, they will need to consider oncoplastic techniques to fill the gap or reshape the breast, or do a mastectomy, with the option of a reconstruction.

Your surgeon will see you in a clinic to give you your results and talk to you about your surgical choices. They may need to examine you again to properly assess your breasts (how firm or droopy they are, whether they are symmetrical) and the quality of your skin. They will also ask you whether you smoke and ask about any other medical conditions. Most people accept the MDT's recommendation, but you can ask to have something different. You may be advised to have a lumpectomy and radiotherapy, but instead choose to have a mastectomy and avoid radiotherapy, like Trish did.

Your surgeon may not be trained to do some or all of the more modern oncoplastic procedures, which means you may need to see a different surgeon if this is something you want to consider.

The key questions you should think about are:

- If you're offered a lumpectomy, would you rather have a mastectomy?
- If you're offered a mastectomy, are there any alternative operations that mean you could keep your breast?
- If you're offered a mastectomy, do you want to stay flat or explore breast reconstruction? (See Chapter 8 for more on this.)

It is your body and your choice. Below, we list some questions to ask yourself – and then (when you've had a think about those) some additional questions to ask your doctor.

Questions to ask yourself
What is your priority?

The most important factor should be getting your cancer treated properly. Although how your breast looks afterwards is important, your life should come before your looks.

Do you know your breasts?

Your breasts are sisters, not twins. One breast is always a bit bigger or droopier than the other. There's no polite way of describing a breast that has 'headed south for winter', but the technical term is 'ptosis'. Your nipples may even be at different heights. Your surgeon will try to match what you already have, but they can never promise perfection.

What do you want to achieve?

Your breasts can define your identity as a woman. You may love them or hate them, wish for bigger or smaller ones, flaunt them or hide them away. They may be incredibly important sexually or they may have very little feeling and you can't see what all the fuss is about. You may have loved your breasts as a young woman, but now you've raised a family, you're not that bothered about them. It's also hard to think rationally about them when you're dealing with a breast cancer diagnosis but knowing how important your breasts are to you can help you decide what to do.

In an ideal world, would you like to look good in clothes, in your bra or naked? You may opt for a quick, simple operation and be happy to wear a small prosthesis in your bra to make you look symmetrical in clothes, or you may choose a longer, more technical operation to try to look symmetrical naked.

Ask your surgeon to show you 'before' and 'after' medical photographs of patients who have had the operation you're considering. If a surgeon shows you a good result and you think it's great, then you're both on the same wavelength. If a surgeon shows you a good result and you think it is awful, you may have to lower your expectations.

Do you mind where the scar is?

If your breast appearance is important to you and you're having a lumpectomy, it's normally possible for your surgeon to hide the scar, for example by placing it at the junction of the nipple–areola complex and the breast. However, this might mean that you lose some nipple sensation. If you're not bothered, they can just cut down directly over the cancer and still leave you with a good result. Breast skin scars can occasionally widen and thicken (hypertrophic scars), and this is more common after a breast reduction. Women of African ancestry are more prone to developing bulky (keloid) scars which extend onto the rest of the breast and can be very difficult to treat. If you have ever developed a thickened scar in the past, mention it to your surgeon.

Do you want to be able to breastfeed in the future?

If you are planning on having children in the future and breast-feeding is important to you, you need to factor this in. You can't breastfeed after a mastectomy because the breast tissue has been removed. Most women can still breastfeed after a lumpectomy unless they have had a breast reduction.

How quickly do you want to get your life back?

If you want to return to work, childcare or sport as quickly as possible you might opt for a simpler operation with a shorter recovery period in order to achieve this. Surgeons initially make decisions based on your tumour size and your breast shape. They tend to want to give you a good cosmetic result as well as removing the cancer, and this may require a lengthy operation with a long recovery period. However, the surgeon isn't the one who has to live with the effects of the surgery, so you need to speak up and let them know what is important to you. Never feel bad about asking for something simpler than the surgeon is proposing.

What will your breast look like in several years' time?

The shape of your operated breast will probably change as the years go by. Radiotherapy fixes a breast in time and place. This means that as your natural breast gets bigger or smaller as you gain or lose weight, or starts to droop as you get older, the cancer side won't change to match it. You may also develop dents in the breast where the cancer was. There are surgical options that you can try to improve the appearance, such as 'lipofilling' (see page 99) and your surgeon will be able to talk to you about them if you are interested in further surgery.

Should you have surgery on your healthy breast?

Removing your healthy breast will not improve your prognosis from breast cancer and it will not stop it coming back in the future. It is the cancer being treated now, not a cancer you might get in years to come, that affects your survival from breast cancer. You should also remember that any chemotherapy or hormonal therapy you have is treating *all* of you, including your healthy breast, which further reduces the chance of you developing a second cancer in your other breast. However, if you have a BRCA mutation, your surgeon may discuss removing your healthy breast because you still have a very high chance of getting a cancer in your other breast in the future.

The other reason to operate on your healthy breast is to make your breasts more symmetrical. If you have large breasts and your surgeon has suggested a breast reduction, you can ask about having a reduction on the other side. While this is a very rewarding operation for both you and your surgeon, it does mean longer surgery with a longer recovery time. Your surgeon will also need to factor in the effects of radiotherapy to the cancer side (which can shrink the treated breast and alter the final appearance), and they may suggest waiting to reduce your normal side until after you have finished radiotherapy. You can wear a small prosthesis in your bra in the meantime.

A small number of women who have had a simple mastectomy ask to have their healthy breast removed for symmetry so they are flat on both sides. Removing healthy tissue is not something that a surgeon will rush into lightly, and it may take many months or years to come to a decision that neither you nor your surgeon will regret in the future. The initial emotions you feel at the time of diagnosis may be completely different to those you feel in six to twelve months' time. Your surgeon may also need to check that they can get the funding to do this on the NHS, as this is technically not a cancer operation.

QUESTIONS TO ASK YOUR SURGEON

- What operation do you recommend, and why?
- Do I definitely need the operation? What happens if I don't have the operation? What are the alternatives?
- How much experience have you had? Have you had oncoplastic training?
- Are there any other operations I could have that you haven't been trained to do that might be suitable?
- Where will the scar be?
- Will I have a drain?
- Can I see photographs of patients who have had the same operation?
- I don't want to have radiotherapy. Can I have a mastectomy instead of a lumpectomy?
- How long will I be in hospital for?
- How long will it take me to get back to normal/recover?
- How much time off work will I need?
- When will I be able to drive?

Why you might not get the result you want

Most surgeons will do everything they can to help you get a good result. Sometimes, though, they need to compromise on the appearance of your breast so they can treat the cancer properly. Smoking and vaping, for example, narrow the blood vessels in your body so your breast and skin don't get as much blood as a person who doesn't smoke. More complex operations, such as a breast reduction, carry a far greater risk of complications and your surgeon might not want to take that chance. If you have medical problems that affect your heart and lungs, such as very high blood pressure or emphysema, the risks from a long general anaesthetic are higher, and your surgeon may guide you towards a quicker, simpler operation.

BREAST OPERATIONS
Lumpectomy (wide local excision)

You will be offered this operation if your cancer is small compared to the size of your breast. An incision is made in the skin, and the cancer is removed with a margin of normal breast tissue. Your surgeon may then move and stitch the remaining breast tissue to close the gap. The skin is normally closed with dissolvable stitches that lie underneath the skin, followed by a waterproof dressing so you can shower afterwards. This is a short operation, and you will go home either the same day or within 24 hours.

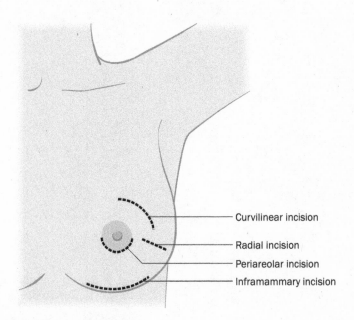

Curvilinear incision

Radial incision

Periareolar incision

Inframammary incision

Examples of lumpectomy scars

Lumpectomy with breast reduction ('therapeutic mammoplasty')

If you have a large cancer in a very large breast, your surgeon can remove up to half of your breast tissue (including the cancer) and skin and reshape the remaining tissue to create a smaller breast.

Your surgeon can't promise you an exact cup size, but most women having breast reduction end up with a C–DD cup. It takes several hours and you may stay in hospital overnight.

There are several different scar patterns. The most common approach is called a 'Wise pattern' which is like an anchor that also goes around the nipple. Most women having this operation lose some or all of their nipple sensation, and there is a small chance that you might lose the nipple itself because of problems with wound healing and poor blood supply. Your breast will be quite swollen for several months afterwards.

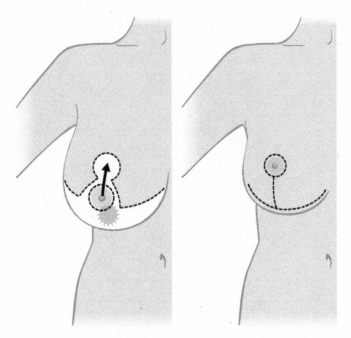

Therapeatic mammoplasty surgery

Lumpectomy with a mini-flap

If you have a large tumour in a small breast, your surgeon can use some of your own tissue (a 'mini-flap') to fill the gap so you don't need a mastectomy. They use fat from either your back (TDAP or Thoracodorsal Artery Perforator flap) or your side (LICAP or

Lateral Intercostal Artery Perforator flap), and you will end up with one long scar extending from the breast onto your chest wall. The operation is sometimes done in two stages. At the first operation, your surgeon simply removes the cancer. Once your results come back and they know that the margins are clear, they will do a second operation a few weeks later to fill the gap in the breast with the flap. This operation takes several hours and has a longer recovery time than a standard lumpectomy. You will be advised not to lift anything heavy for two to three months, and this might not be practical if you are very active or have small children.

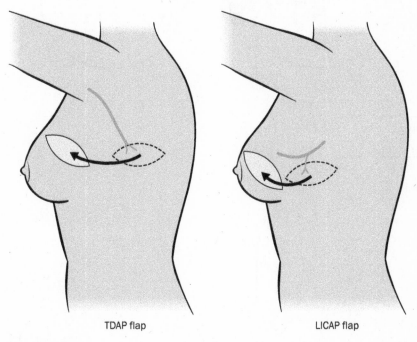

TDAP flap   LICAP flap

Mini-flap surgery

Lumpectomy for cancers involving or close to the nipple

If your cancer involves the nipple or lies directly beneath it, your nipple has to be removed as part of the cancer operation. If your breasts are large enough, your surgeon might be able to rotate some of your breast tissue and skin to fill the gap, followed by a nipple reconstruction at a later date if you want one (see Chapter 8 for more on this). If you have small breasts, you can either have a lumpectomy (leaving you with a scar in the middle of your breast where your nipple was), or a mastectomy with a reconstruction if you prefer.

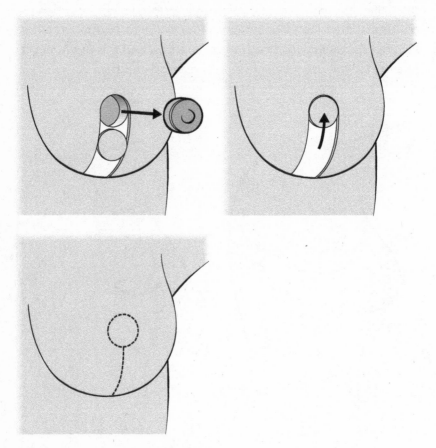

Surgery for cancer behind the nipple

Mastectomy

A mastectomy means removing all of your breast tissue together with the breast skin and nipple, leaving you with a low, curved scar on your chest wall. Your surgeon will try to streamline the scar, but you may be left with a small 'dog-ear' that can be neatened up at a smaller operation in the future. The skin is normally closed with dissolvable stitches that lie underneath the skin, with a waterproof dressing on top. Many women have a 'cuddly bit' at the edge of the breast that blends into the skin and fat of your back that you don't normally see because the breast hides it. When the breast tissue is removed, it may be very noticeable when you look in the mirror.

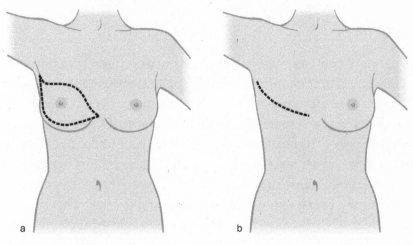

Mastectomy surgery

After your mastectomy, you will be given a soft cotton temporary prosthesis to put in your bra until the skin underneath has fully healed. This can move around because it is so light, so you may want to use a safety pin to attach it to your bra. After six to eight weeks, your breast care nurse will arrange for you to be fitted for a more permanent prosthesis. These are made of silicone, and come in different shapes, sizes and colour tones, with or without a nipple. If you were treated privately, you may have to pay for a prosthesis from a department store or specialist supplier. Alternatively, you could ask your GP to refer you to an NHS prosthetic fitting service at your local breast unit.

SIDE EFFECTS AND COMPLICATIONS AFTER BREAST SURGERY

Some complications, such as loss of nipple sensation and asymmetry between your breasts, are unavoidable because of the techniques your surgeon uses. Asymmetry can develop several months or years later because of radiotherapy, weight loss/gain and the ageing process.

Seroma

The most common side effect after breast surgery is a seroma. This is a collection of tissue fluid in the space where you had your surgery, and the fluid does not contain cancer cells. Everybody produces some seroma fluid which is normally absorbed over several weeks. You may, however, produce a lot of fluid which can make your breast feel tight and uncomfortable. If this happens to you, tell your breast care nurse and they will arrange to drain the fluid in the breast clinic using a needle and syringe. This doesn't normally hurt, because they drain the seroma through the scar which is numb.

Wound infection

There is a small chance that you will get a wound infection. The risk is greater if you are having more complex surgery, such as a breast reduction, or if you have diabetes or smoke. You may be given a short course of antibiotics to reduce the risk of you getting an infection.

Bleeding

There is a small chance that you might bleed after the operation. This can happen in the first couple of hours after you wake up and may mean you will need another small operation to stop the bleeding. Alternatively, you might develop a blood clot inside the breast over the next couple of days. This can usually be drained in the clinic, but you might need another small operation to remove it.

Pain

If you have a mastectomy, there is a small (15–30 per cent) chance that you will be left with chronic pain after your operation, and this can be permanent. It is called post-mastectomy pain syndrome (PMPS) and we don't know why it happens. You may have a burning or a tingling sensation in the skin on the chest wall and upper arm. There are several different types of painkillers that can be used to treat this, and your surgeon and GP will be able to help you.

ARMPIT OPERATIONS

Your armpit is also called your 'axilla'. You will be advised to have one of two operations, depending on the results of your triple assessment (see Chapter 2 and page 11).

Sentinel node biopsy

If the ultrasound scan of your armpit was normal, your surgeon will remove the first node that breast cancer spreads to (the sentinel node) to make sure that it doesn't contain cancer cells. Even though your nodes looked normal on the scan, there is still a 20–30 per cent chance that there might be tiny cancer deposits which are too small to see.

Two techniques are used to find the sentinel node (some surgeons use just one and some use both together). The first technique uses a small amount of a radioactive tracer liquid which is injected into your breast, normally on the day of your operation. The liquid gets trapped in the sentinel node and your surgeon uses a probe to find it. You are not radioactive after the operation, and it is safe for you to be around your family. The total amount of radiation that you receive is tiny (less than you get from the environment over a three-month period).

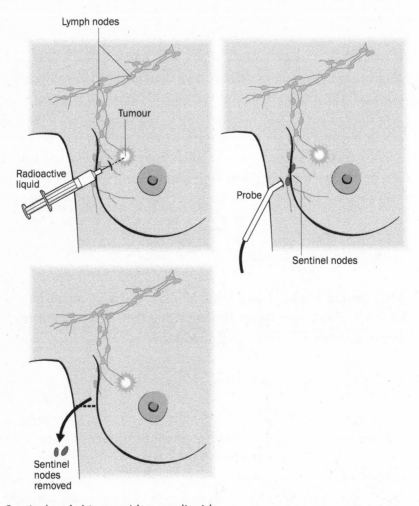

Sentinel node biopsy with tracer liquid

The second technique uses a small amount of blue dye which is injected near your nipple while you are asleep. This fluid is also carried in the lymph vessels to the nodes and stains them blue so your surgeon can easily see them. Your surgeon removes all the radioactive nodes and/or all the blue nodes – normally one to three in total.

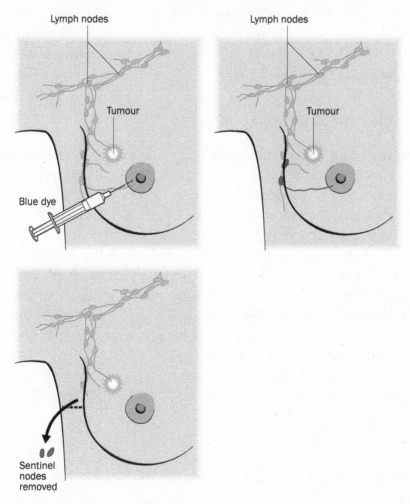

Sentinel node biopsy with blue dye

Newer techniques are being introduced, such as magnetic microscopic beads and fluorescent dyes. Your surgeon will explain these to you if they plan to use them.

The sentinel node biopsy is normally done through a small scar just below the hairline in your armpit, but sometimes your surgeon can remove the node through your breast scar. If you are having a mastectomy, the surgeon will use the mastectomy scar to remove the node.

Some breast units have a machine that can analyse your sentinel node for cancer cells in real time while you're having your operation (OSNA, or One Step Nucleic Acid Amplification). If the node is positive, your surgeon can remove the rest of your armpit lymph nodes while you are still asleep, instead of having another operation a few weeks later.

Axillary node clearance

If your triple assessment showed that you have cancer cells in your lymph nodes, your surgeon will remove most of the lymph nodes in your armpit. This is called an axillary node clearance. There are three levels of nodes in your axilla. Level I nodes are low in your armpit, Level II nodes are higher up, and Level III nodes are higher still, next to the major blood vessels and nerves that supply your arm. Your surgeon will normally remove all the nodes in Levels I and II (10–20 in total). Level III nodes are not routinely removed because of the much higher risk of developing side effects, such as lymphoedema (see page 96) and because removing these nodes does not improve your prognosis.

The axillary node clearance operation is done through a scar below the hairline in your armpit. If you are having a mastectomy, it is done through the breast scar.

SIDE EFFECTS AND COMPLICATIONS AFTER ARMPIT SURGERY

Seromas, wound infections and bleeding (described on pages 90 and 91) can also occur in the armpit. You will probably be told not to lift anything heavy for the first couple of weeks, to allow the wound to heal and reduce the chance of these problems occurring.

After-effects of the dye

If you have a sentinel node biopsy, the skin around your nipple will be stained blue from the dye. This normally fades over a few months, but it can last for up to a year. The dye may also turn your urine

Trish developed a small seroma in her armpit following her sentinel node biopsy. She had it drained twice but the fluid reaccumulated each time. Many months later, the seroma became infected (possibly because her immune system was low due to chemotherapy) and had to be drained in an operation. It took several weeks to heal but eventually Trish's armpit felt normal again.

blue-green for a day or two, but this is nothing to worry about. There is a very, very small chance (2 in every 1,000 patients) of developing a serious allergic reaction to the blue dye, which normally happens during the operation while you are still asleep and can usually be treated with anti-allergy drugs, such as steroids and antihistamines.

Numbness

After either operation, you may notice a patch of skin on your upper inner arm that feels numb, like 'pins and needles'. There is a nerve that runs between the nodes in your armpit which provides sensation to that patch of skin. Sometimes your surgeon has to stretch the nerve or cut it during surgery, and this causes the numbness. If the nerve was stretched, then the feeling will return over time. If the nerve is cut, then that patch of skin will be permanently numb.

In addition to the above, there are three specific complications following armpit surgery that can affect the use of your arm: shoulder stiffness, lymphoedema and cording. The risk of getting any of these is higher after an axillary clearance.

Shoulder stiffness

Your shoulder will feel sore and stiff after your operation. You should have been given a series of exercises to do that can also be found on the Breast Cancer Care website (see page 277). These start gently and build up as you get more movement in your arm.

It is really important that you do them at least three times a day to help you get your movement and function back.

You may still have a stiff shoulder despite doing the exercises, and occasionally this can turn into a 'frozen shoulder'. If your pain and stiffness isn't getting better, you should see your GP. They may need to refer you to a physiotherapist or orthopaedic surgeon for further treatment.

Lymphoedema

Lymphoedema is when fluid collects in the soft tissues of your arm (and sometimes your breast) because the lymph vessels were cut during surgery when your surgeon removed the nodes, which causes your hand and arm to swell. After a sentinel node biopsy, your risk is 5–10 per cent (1 in 10–20) in your lifetime. After an axillary clearance, your risk is 25 per cent (1 in 4). It can take several years to develop, and there is no cure, which means that once you develop it, you will always have a swollen arm.

Your breast care nurse will tell you what signs to look out for, and there is detailed information on the Macmillan and Breast Cancer Care websites (see page 277). The first signs are swelling, tightness or discomfort in your fingers and hand, such as a ring or watch strap feeling tight, or long-sleeved clothing becoming hard to get on. If this happens, you should contact your breast care nurse who will refer you to your local lymphoedema unit.

To reduce your risk of developing lymphoedema, you should use your arm normally and continue to do your shoulder exercises. Regular exercise, such as swimming and walking, will help. Try to avoid gaining a lot of weight, as this increases the pressure on the lymphatic system and can lead to the development of lymphoedema.

There is no hard evidence to say that having blood or your blood pressure taken from your 'at risk' arm will definitely increase the risk of you developing lymphoedema. However, most doctors will still advise you to use the other arm where possible. Keep your arm moisturised, and use strong sunscreen on holiday, as sunburn can also increase the risk of developing lymphoedema.

After armpit surgery, you are more likely to get an infection in your hand or arm following a small cut or graze because you have fewer nodes to fight infection. This infection can then spread and become serious. The infection can also increase the risk of you getting lymphoedema. Use simple precautions like wearing gloves when gardening, using clean, fresh razors when shaving your underarms, and keep any cuts or grazes clean. If you think you might have an infection (the cut looks red, hot, swollen or is painful), see your GP immediately as you may need antibiotics.

Lymphoedema is treated in three ways: massage, compression and surgery. Massage involves a special technique called manual lymphatic drainage (MLD) to slowly move the fluid away from your swollen arm. It must be done by a trained lymphoedema therapist. They may teach you to do MLD yourself. The second

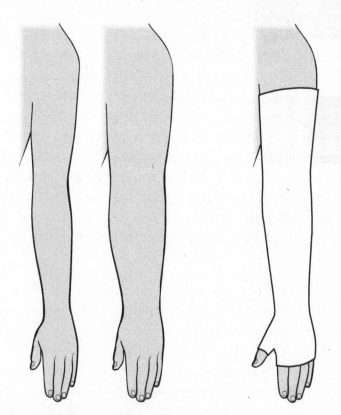

Lymphoedema and a compression sleeve

treatment involves wearing a compression glove or a sleeve for the rest of your life, which reduces and prevents further swelling. The ones issued free on the NHS are skin tone in colour, but you can buy patterned ones online. New surgical techniques have recently been developed in Europe where lymph nodes from other areas in your body, such as your groin, are transplanted into your arm. These transplanted nodes are then able to help drain the fluid from your swollen arm. This operation may soon be available in the UK.

Cording (axillary web syndrome)

You could develop tight, rope-like structures called 'cords' that run from your armpit scar down your inner upper arm. Your arm will feel painful and tight, and the cords stop you being able to fully move your shoulder and get your arm above your head. We still don't know why they form.

The first treatment is to continue with your shoulder exercises as the cords will often snap by themselves as you stretch your arm. This isn't painful. You may feel a 'pinging' sensation or even hear a pop as they snap, followed by relief as you can suddenly move your arm. Lying on the side of your bed and letting your arm hang off the edge is often very effective, as gravity helps you get a better stretch.

When you have radiotherapy, you have to lie with your arms above your head so your breasts are in the right position to be treated. If cording means that you can't get your arms above your head, your radiotherapy will need to be delayed. You may need to see a physiotherapist to help massage the area and snap the cords.

Cording happened to Liz, whose radiotherapy was delayed by three months as a result. Despite doing all the stretching exercises she still couldn't get her arm above her head. After two sessions with a trained physiotherapist, she could fully move her arm again.

ADDITIONAL SURGERY

Re-excision of margins

Your surgeon removes all the cancer they can feel, but sometimes there may be cells close to the margins that can only be seen with a microscope (in other words, you have a 'positive margin'). Up to 4 in every 10 women need further surgery to get a clear margin. In rare cases, you may even need a third operation if the margins still aren't clear. If you have small breasts or have had a breast reduction, your surgeon may need to do a mastectomy to get clear margins.

Completion axillary node clearance

If your sentinel node biopsy was positive, your surgeon will discuss further treatment to the axilla. This may be a completion axillary node clearance, or radiotherapy (see Chapter 12) to the armpit at the same time as your breast radiotherapy.

Lipofilling

If you have a visible defect after your surgery or radiotherapy and have enough fat, your surgeon can use your own fat to fill in the defect. Fat is harvested from your tummy or thighs, cleaned and then injected into the breast. You may need several operations to get a good result. Lipofilling does not increase the risk of the cancer coming back.

Surgery for a local recurrence

If your cancer comes back as a nodule in the skin, your surgeon will remove the nodule with a rim of normal tissue around it. If your cancer comes back in your breast after a lumpectomy, your only option is a mastectomy. This is because you have already had radiotherapy, and you cannot have radiotherapy again.

Surgery to the breast and armpit is quite complicated as every breast is different and every patient is different, so there is no 'one-size-fits-all' operation. We hope that you've now got a better understanding of why your surgeon has recommended a specific operation to you.

If you need to have a mastectomy, your surgeon should talk to you about having your breast reconstructed. This is even more complicated and can take two or three consultations with your medical team to come to a final decision. We guide you through all the various options in the next chapter to help you decide what to do.

CHAPTER 8

BREAST RECONSTRUCTION

A BREAST RECONSTRUCTION is an operation to recreate a breast shape after a mastectomy. Your surgeon will try to match your opposite breast size and shape. There are two ways to do this. The first uses a breast implant, and the second uses your own fat and muscle (called a 'flap' or 'autologous' reconstruction). Your reconstruction may be done at the same time as your mastectomy, or many months or years later.

DO YOU WANT A BREAST RECONSTRUCTION?

When you hear that you need a mastectomy, your initial reaction may be shock, fear or even horror. This is completely normal. Most of us rarely think about what our breasts mean to us, and it's even harder to think about them with regards to sexuality and body image when your judgement is clouded by the fact that you've been told that you have breast cancer. You might think that having a mastectomy means you'll lose your confidence, femininity and sexuality but this isn't necessarily true, and many women choose to stay flat-chested after surgery. However, having a breast reconstruction can boost your self-esteem and help you feel feminine and confident, especially if your breasts are important to you. There is nothing wrong with being concerned about your appearance, and having a reconstruction does not mean you are being vain.

If you do need to have a mastectomy, your surgeon should discuss breast reconstruction with you when they are planning that first operation. Not every breast surgeon is trained to do every type of reconstruction, but they should talk to you about all of the available options, even if it means another surgeon does your reconstruction at another hospital. It is important to discuss your thoughts and feelings, especially with your partner (if you have one), but ultimately it is your body and your decision to make. There are patients who decide to have a reconstruction to keep their partner, or even their surgeon, happy, and live to regret it, especially if they end up having a complication that needs further operations to fix it. We urge you not to do something just to make other people happy.

WHAT IS ACHIEVABLE?

Every surgeon wants to give you a great result but they can't promise perfection. It helps if you can decide whether your priority is to look good in your clothes, in your bra or naked. This will guide your surgeon and they can then be realistic about what is achievable. If you have an implant, your reconstructed breast won't age like your natural breast (which changes in size and shape and starts to droop as you get older). The great result you have in the first year after your surgery may not look quite as good in the future. Radiotherapy can also affect the shape of a reconstruction, especially if you have an implant (see page 111 for more information), and your surgeon will talk to you about this in more detail.

Your new breast won't feel like your healthy breast when someone touches it. This is because the nerves in your skin and nipple are cut when your breast tissue is removed. You may only feel a pins and needles sensation when your breast is touched, or you might not feel anything at all. You won't get a sexual response when your breast or nipple is stimulated.

Why you might not get your ideal reconstruction

There are several reasons why your surgeon may not be able to give you your ideal reconstruction:

Do you have the right breast and body shape?

If you want to use your own tissue, you need to have enough of it to recreate a breast. If you are very thin, you are unlikely to have enough body fat and muscle for a flap-based reconstruction. It is also impossible to recreate a large, droopy breast using an implant unless you have a breast reduction on the other side.

Both Trish and Liz were advised to have implants because they didn't have enough tissue for a flap-based reconstruction.

Are you fit enough?

If you have other medical conditions, such as very high blood pressure, it might not be medically safe for you to have the longer general anaesthetic that a reconstruction needs (the operation can take up to six to eight hours). Although age per se should not be a barrier to reconstruction surgery, your surgeon does need to be frank with you about how the operation might affect you. It takes much longer to recover from a major operation if you are in your sixties and seventies, and you may never fully 'bounce back' to the person you were before.

Do you smoke/use e-cigarettes?

The nicotine in cigarettes narrows the blood vessels in the body. When you have a mastectomy, the blood supply to the breast skin is reduced because your breast tissue has been removed. Smoking reduces the blood supply to the skin even more, and there is a high chance that your scars won't heal. To fix this, your surgeon would probably need to remove the reconstruction (leaving you with a flat chest). Some animal studies have shown that vaping and e-cigarettes also cause problems with wound healing. Many surgeons won't take that risk and will recommend that you have a mastectomy to treat your cancer, followed by a delayed reconstruction after you have stopped smoking.

How long do you want to take to recover?

It takes a couple of months to recover from implant surgery, and up to six months to recover from flap surgery, compared to a couple of weeks following a simple mastectomy. If you can't (or don't want to) put your life on hold to recover from surgery – for example, if you have young children to look after or elderly relatives to care for – you may need to compromise on the look and feel of your new breast (choosing an implant with a shorter recovery time), or delay your reconstruction until you're ready for it.

WHERE CAN YOU GET HELP TO MAKE A DECISION?

When your surgeon first talks to you about reconstruction, you will be given information about the different options. This may be a lot to take on board, especially when you're still dealing with a new breast cancer diagnosis. It can help to talk to other women who have had a reconstruction, and your breast care nurse will know if there is a local support group where you can meet patient volunteers. You can also talk to other patients in forums on websites such as Breast Cancer Care and Macmillan. Breast Cancer Care has an animated guide on their website. The Touch Surgery app may also be useful. It is designed for trainee surgeons and shows surgical details of the operations, so is quite graphic. (See the Resources section on page 276 for more details.)

CAN YOU HAVE A BREAST RECONSTRUCTION IF YOU HAVE SECONDARY BREAST CANCER?

If you have secondary breast cancer when you are diagnosed, or have had a mastectomy and developed metastases before your delayed reconstruction, you may still be able to have a breast reconstruction. Most surgeons will want to make sure that your cancer has been stable for a minimum of three months, i.e. your scans haven't shown any new deposits, and your current metastases haven't increased in size. You also need to be strong enough to cope with, and recover from, a big operation, and it will need to fit around your ongoing cancer treatment.

PLANNING YOUR BREAST RECONSTRUCTION

Your surgeon will help you decide when to have your reconstruction. There are two options:

1. *Immediate reconstruction* happens at the same time as your mastectomy. It gives the best cosmetic results because the surgeon can put the implant or flap inside your natural breast skin. There is also the psychological boost of never having a flat chest or having to wear a false breast (prosthesis) in your bra.
2. *Delayed reconstruction* happens months to years after your mastectomy. This could be due to personal preference, being pregnant when you are diagnosed or your doctors advising you to wait until after you've finished other treatments, such as chemotherapy and radiotherapy. The cosmetic result from a delayed reconstruction is often not as good as an immediate reconstruction. Because your breast skin has been removed, your surgeon needs to stretch the remaining skin with an expander implant (if you haven't had radiotherapy) or use skin from your flap to help recreate a breast shape. If they use skin from your flap, you will have a scar that goes all the way around your new breast, instead of a small scar in the middle or at the side.

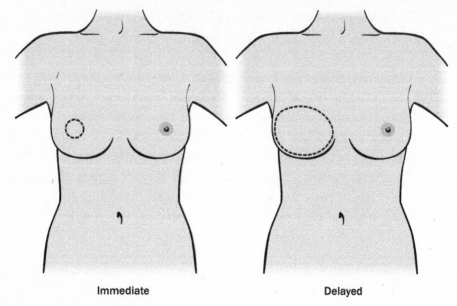

Immediate   Delayed

Breast reconstruction scars

What is the difference between an implant and a flap-based reconstruction?

The first difference is the feel of the new breast. An implant feels like a soft, firm bag of jelly. It doesn't move when you run or jump. It will always look 'perky' while your natural breast will change shape with time. Implants are best suited for women with small A–D cup breasts that aren't droopy. A flap-based reconstruction uses your own tissue and it looks, feels and moves like your other breast. This is a good option if you have small breasts and want to avoid an implant, or have large or droopy breasts and don't want to make your breasts smaller (provided you have enough tissue to use).

The second major difference is the surgery and recovery time. Implant surgery is relatively quick (2–4 hours), involves a short stay in hospital (usually 1–3 nights) and a 1–2-month recovery period. There is only one scar (the mastectomy scar on the breast). The natural lifespan of an implant is 10–15 years, and you may want or need to have further surgery in the future to revise the shape and feel of the implant (especially if you have radiotherapy), or to reshape the other breast to maintain symmetry.

Flap-based surgery, on the other hand, involves a much longer operation (5–10 hours), a 3–7-night stay in hospital and a 3–6-month recovery period. You have at least two scars, which means double the risk of a wound complication. You may want or need a second shorter operation to tidy up the scars, boost the shape with lipofilling (see page 99) and create a new nipple to get the best cosmetic outcome.

Do you need to see a plastic surgeon?

Most consultant breast surgeons are trained to do implant reconstructions, and some do back- and tummy-based flap-based reconstructions as well. Plastic surgeons are trained to do all the flap-based reconstructions. If your breast surgeon isn't trained to do the reconstruction that you prefer, they will refer you to see a plastic surgeon who will do your operation. The plastic surgeon may work in a different hospital. Your breast surgeon would then travel to that hospital to do your mastectomy while the plastic surgeon does the flap.

Being examined by a plastic surgeon can feel quite impersonal. This is because they have to look at your body for muscle and fat that could be used to recreate a breast, and this means examining your tummy, thigh, bottom and lower back fat. It can feel embarrassing to stand there in your knickers while the surgeon grabs a handful of tummy fat, but it is the only way to work out whether you have enough tissue to recreate a breast.

Can your breasts be made bigger or smaller at the same time?

If you have very large breasts, it may be possible to make both breasts smaller at the same time by doing a breast reduction (see page 78). If you used to have large breasts that have now 'deflated' a bit (perhaps after pregnancy), your surgeon may be able to give you fuller breasts. However, if you are naturally small-breasted, it is difficult for your surgeon to make your breasts larger. This is because your breast skin has to be able to stretch to accommodate the implant or tissue being used. If the skin is stretched too much, like an elastic band about to snap, it may start to die in places. This can leave holes in the skin or a scar that won't heal. If this happens, your surgeon will have to remove the reconstruction and leave you with a flat chest while everything heals, and this could delay chemotherapy or radiotherapy.

Can you keep your nipple?

Whether you can keep your nipple depends on the position of the cancer in your breast and the size of your breast. If the cancer involves or lies directly behind your nipple, your surgeon must remove the nipple when they do the mastectomy.

If the cancer isn't close to the nipple, you may be able to keep your nipple. This does slightly increase the risk of getting a recurrence in the breast, but the overall risk of recurrence after a mastectomy is still very low. Your surgeon may want to take a biopsy from behind your nipple first to make sure that the nipple doesn't contain cancer cells.

In order to keep your nipple, your surgeon has to make sure it will get enough blood from your breast skin to survive. If it doesn't get enough blood, it may start to die and even fall off, leaving you with a flat stump. The larger your breasts, the further the blood has to travel to reach the nipple and the more likely it is to die. As a general rule, if your breasts are larger than a D cup, your nipple is less likely to survive.

If you can't keep your nipple, you may be able to have a nipple reconstruction later. The nipple is normally made using a flap of skin from the middle of your reconstruction using a local anaesthetic and takes about 20 minutes. Many women have it tattooed (often by breast care nurses) to make it look more realistic. If you don't want another operation, you can

Liz's cancer was in the top half of her breast, and she chose to have a nipple-sparing mastectomy. The nipple looked a bit battered and bruised for a few weeks, and then the tip became scabby and fell off (a bit like when a baby's umbilical cord falls off). This didn't hurt, but it was a bit 'gross'! She was left with a flat nipple stump.

Trish's cancer involved her nipple, so she couldn't keep it. Six months after her initial implant surgery, she had a new nipple (which sticks up like her normal nipple) made using the skin of her reconstructed breast. This took about 20 minutes, using a local anaesthetic. She decided not to have a nipple tattoo to make it look more realistic, but knows she can have it done in the future.

either have a nipple tattoo without a nipple reconstruction, or use a stick-on silicone nipple.

Do you need to buy a special bra to wear after your reconstruction?

Most surgeons will ask you to wear a bra day and night for the first 2–4 weeks after your reconstruction. This helps support the new breast and can ease discomfort. Ideally you want a post-mastectomy bra, with a front fastening, so it is easy to get on and off, and a range of fastenings to allow for post-op swelling. You can buy a post-mastectomy bra from most high street stores and even supermarkets, although they may not cater for women with a very small or large bra size. You could also try online specialist mastectomy bra retailers such as Amoena and Nicola Jane, and companies like Recoheart and Macom that only sell post-surgery bras (see page 280–1 for details). Your breast care nurse will also be able to advise you.

QUESTIONS TO ASK YOUR SURGEON

Breast reconstruction is complicated and there are many things to take into account. The following questions may help you as you plan your discussion with your surgeon:

- Can I have a reconstruction?
- What's the difference between an implant and a flap-based reconstruction? Are both these options available for me?
- What kind of reconstruction would give me the best shape?
- Should I have my reconstruction at the same time as my mastectomy or wait until after I've finished treatment?
- If I want to go flat now, can I have a reconstruction in the future?
- Can you make my breasts bigger (or smaller) while you are doing the reconstruction?
- Can I keep my nipple?
- Where will the scars be?
- Where will I have the operation?
- How long will the surgery take?
- How long will I be in hospital for?
- Do I need to wear a special bra afterwards?
- How long will it take me to recover and get back to my normal activities?
- What are the complications?
- What happens if it goes wrong?
- What will it look and feel like in the months and years ahead?
- What experience do you have in this operation?
- Can I see photos of your patients who have had this reconstruction? (All medical photos are anonymous and don't show patients' heads.)
- Can I talk to a patient who has had this operation?

IMPLANT RECONSTRUCTION

A permanent breast implant is a strong silicone shell filled with silicone that comes in a wide variety of shapes and sizes so the surgeon can match your opposite breast volume, height and width. Implants undergo rigorous laboratory testing and have to be approved by the Medicines & Healthcare products Regulatory Agency (MRHA) which ensures that they are safe and fit for use. It is almost impossible to damage an implant. If you have an implant in the UK, you will be asked if your details can be stored in the NHS Breast and Cosmetic Implant Registry. This means that any problems with your implant can be carefully followed up, and it is easier for research to be done looking at implant complications in the future.

A temporary implant is also called a 'tissue expander'. This is an empty silicone shell that can be filled with sterile water. Some tissue expanders have a small amount of silicone inside them as well. They are filled up using a port, which is located either in the middle of the implant or connected via a small plastic tube which sits at your bra line.

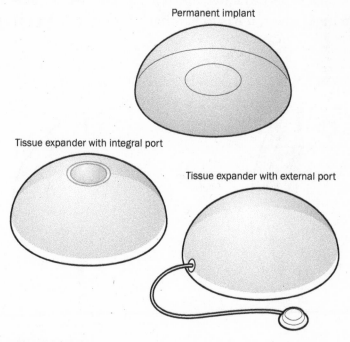

Permanent implant

Tissue expander with integral port

Tissue expander with external port

Types of breast implant

What is the difference between a one-stage and two-stage operation?

There are several different ways to reconstruct a breast using an implant, and they can all give good results. Every surgeon has their preferred technique. A one-stage operation means that your surgeon puts in a permanent implant at the same time as the reconstruction. A two-stage operation means that your surgeon first uses a tissue expander, which is slowly expanded every couple of weeks in clinic. Once the expander has reached the right size for you, your surgeon will swap it for a permanent implant at a second operation, normally three to six months later. This is often done if you need to have radiotherapy.

What happens during surgery?

The implant has to be completely covered by tissue, and this can be done in one of two ways. The first uses your chest muscle (pectoralis major) to cover the implant. Because the muscle lies flat on your chest, it has to be stretched using a tissue expander.

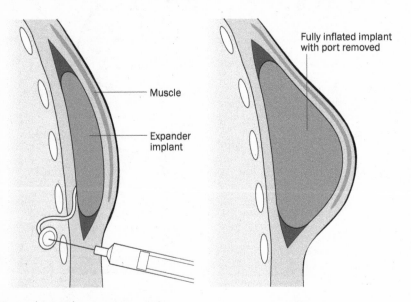

Fully inflated implant with port removed

Muscle

Expander implant

Expander implant reconstruction

The expander is slowly filled with sterile water in the outpatient clinic. This gradually stretches the muscle until the right breast size is reached. At a second operation, your surgeon will either remove the port and leave the expander implant in place, or swap it for a permanent silicone implant.

The second technique uses a special mesh called an acellular dermal matrix (ADM) to cover some or all of the silicone implant, and this often gives your reconstruction a more natural shape. There are two ways to use the mesh. The first way (sub-pectoral) involves lifting the chest muscle, putting the top half of the implant underneath it and then sewing a mesh from the bottom of the muscle to your chest wall at the bra line to create a sling for the lower half of the implant.

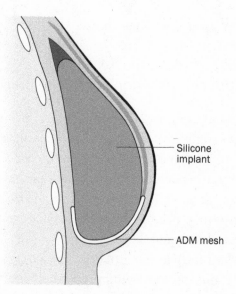

Silicone implant

ADM mesh

Sub-pectoral implant/mesh reconstruction

The second way (pre-pectoral) involves covering the implant completely in mesh and stitching this mesh on top of the muscle.

Your surgeon will tell you which method will give you the best result. If you have an implant, you will probably have one or two drains (see page 128) which are left in for several days to stop fluid building up around the implant which can delay healing.

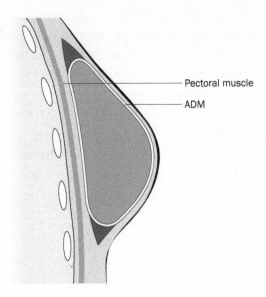

Pectoral muscle

ADM

Pre-pectoral implant/mesh reconstruction

What are the complications of implant reconstruction?

On top of the complications from a simple mastectomy (see page 90), there are complications specific to implant surgery. There is a greater risk of a wound infection because your surgeon is putting a foreign object inside you, and you will probably be given antibiotics to take at home to prevent this. If you do develop a wound infection, you may need to have the implant removed, let everything settle and try again later.

If your chest muscle was lifted during surgery, you may notice that the implant appears to jump up when you flex that muscle. This can be hard to fix, and is more noticeable in slim women.

Your body forms a shell around the implant called a 'capsule' which is normally thin and can't be seen or felt. Over time (months or years), the capsule can thicken and cause visible ripples or folds underneath the skin. It can also contract and change the shape of the implant, or cause pain. Radiotherapy increases the likelihood of this happening. If this happens to you,

114

your surgeon may recommend an operation to release or remove the capsule and replace the implant together with lipofilling (see page 99) to smooth out any visible ripples.

A very rare but serious complication of implant surgery is the development of a rare cancer called Breast Implant-Associated Anaplastic Large Cell Lymphoma (BIA-ALCL). This is a form of non-Hodgkin Lymphoma, a cancer of white blood cells. The risk of developing this is less than 1 in 6,000 women, and may be linked to implants with a textured surface. It typically develops several years after your surgery, and the main symptom is a swollen breast. If caught early, it is treated with surgery and has a very good prognosis.

FLAP-BASED RECONSTRUCTION

A flap is some of your own tissue (fat, muscle or fat and muscle) that is used to reconstruct your breast. The area it is taken from is called the 'donor site'. There are two types of flaps:

1. *Pedicled flaps* stay attached to the donor site (e.g. upper back and tummy) and are rotated to reach your chest wall and create a breast shape.
2. *Free flaps* are disconnected from the donor site (e.g. tummy, lower back, thigh and bottom) and their blood vessels are carefully plumbed into blood vessels on your chest wall using a microscope.

Sometimes your surgeon needs to use a small implant to match the volume of your opposite breast. You will have at least two scars: one on the breast and one or more at the donor site. Your surgeon will probably leave a plastic tube called a drain at the donor site to remove any fluid that collects there (see page 128).

The flap or donor tissue can come from your upper or lower back, tummy, thigh or bottom.

Upper back (latissimus dorsi (LD) flap)

This is a pedicle flap that uses a large back muscle called latissimus dorsi with fat from your upper back. You have a scar on your back where your bra sits. You may have some back and shoulder weakness which should improve in time as other muscles learn to make up for the missing muscle. If you play a lot of sport, this might not be the best choice for you.

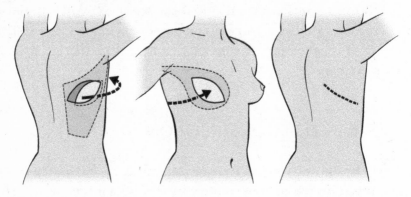

LD flap reconstruction

Lower back (lumbar artery perforator (LAP) flap)

This is a free flap that uses your 'love handles'. You will have a scar on your lower back, normally below your waistline.

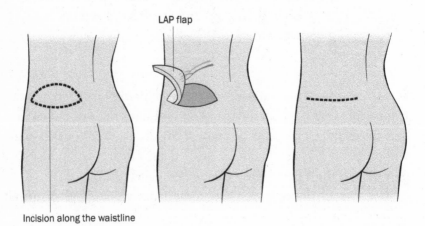

LAP flap

Incision along the waistline

LAP flap reconstruction

Tummy (tranverse rectus abdominus muscle (TRAM) flap)

This is either a pedicle or a free flap that uses a muscle from your tummy called the rectus abdominus muscle together with some overlying fat. You have a low scar on your tummy that goes from hip to hip. You will have a weak core because you have lost one of the muscles that helps you pull your tummy in.

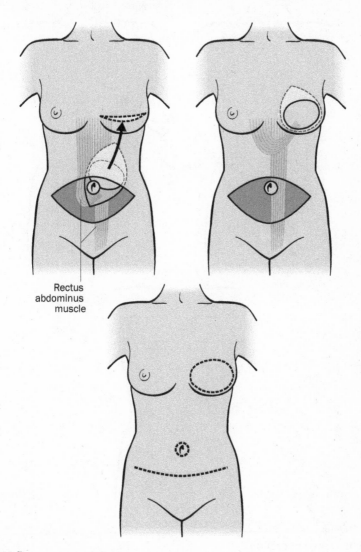

Rectus
abdominus
muscle

TRAM flap reconstruction

Tummy (deep inferior epigastric perforator (DIEP) flap)

This is a free flap that uses your tummy fat below your belly button. It gets its blood supply from a vessel called the deep inferior epigastric perforator. It is essentially a 'tummy tuck' but instead of being

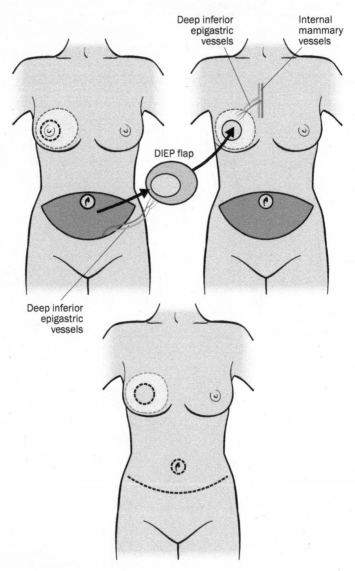

DIEP flap reconstruction

thrown away, the fat is used to make a breast. You are left with a long, low scar going from hip to hip.

Thigh (transverse upper gracilis (TUG) flap)

This is a free flap that uses the gracilis muscle in your inner thigh and your inner thigh fat 'roll'. The other muscles in your leg make up for the one that is used in the reconstruction. The scar runs all the way around your inner upper thigh at the groin, from front to back. If you are slender, you may need the muscles from both thighs to get the necessary volume.

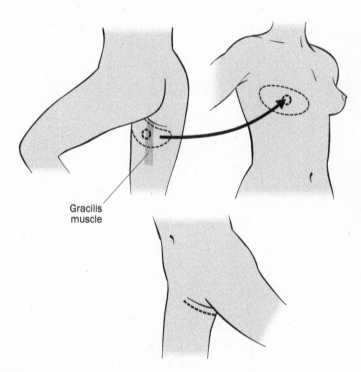

Gracilis
muscle

TUG flap reconstruction

Thigh (profunda artery perforator (PAP) flap)

This is very similar to the TUG flap, but only uses fat from the back of your upper thigh, just underneath your buttock.

Thigh (lateral perforator flap)

This is a free flap that uses the fat 'roll' on your outer thigh, with a scar on the outside of your thigh, below your hip.

Bottom (superior (or inferior) gluteal artery perforator (SGAP/IGAP) flap)

This is a free flap using fat from your upper or lower buttock to recreate the breast. One of the downsides is that you end up with a flatter bottom on that side.

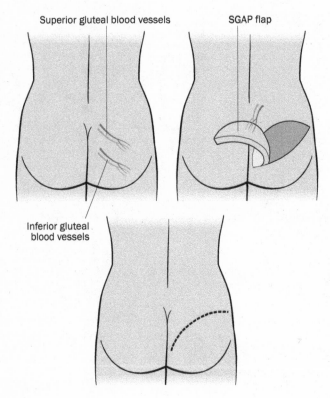

SGAP flap reconstruction

What are the complications of flap reconstruction?

As well as complications from your mastectomy (see page 90), you could have any of those complications at your donor site. These include problems with wound healing, fluid collection (seroma), bleeding and infection. You may also notice weakness at your donor site, especially if a muscle was used to reconstruct your breast.

It is normal for some of the fat at the edges of your reconstructed breast to die away because it isn't getting enough blood. This may cause a hard, lumpy area, or you may notice a dimple or a dent in your new breast. The fat can be replaced with lipofilling at a second operation (see page 99).

Finally, there is a very small chance that your flap doesn't work. This is normally because it isn't getting enough blood, possibly because of a blood clot in one of the blood vessels. Your surgeon may be able to fix this at a second operation, but a very small number of women may end up flat-chested.

As you can see, deciding whether to have a breast reconstruction involves a lot of careful thinking and planning by both you and your surgeon, so you get the best possible outcome. However, the operation itself can be daunting, and in the next chapter we're going to walk you through what happens on the day of your operation, what you need to take with you, and share our tips to help you recover afterwards.

CHAPTER 9

HAVING AN OPERATION

YOU MAY WELL have had an operation before, but if it's the first time you've had one this basic introduction may be helpful. Having an operation is the same as having surgery. Your surgeon will make an incision (a cut) in your skin, use instruments to remove your breast cancer or lymph nodes, and will then stitch the skin closed.

Why do you need an operation?

Surgery is the main treatment for breast cancer. It also allows your doctors to get more information about what type of breast cancer you have and whether your lymph nodes are involved so they can plan what further treatment you might need.

Where do you have your operation?

Your surgery is done in an operating theatre, which is a specially designed room that has all the equipment that your surgeon and anaesthetist need, and is kept spotlessly clean. It is in a separate part of the hospital from the wards and the clinics, with a recovery area next to it where you will wake up. As well as your surgeon, anaesthetist and their trainees, there are also surgical nurses and healthcare practitioners in the theatre who help with your operation.

Who will do your operation?

In the NHS, your consultant surgeon (a surgeon who has finished their training) works with junior doctors who are training to become a consultant. These trainees may do some or all of your operation, under the supervision of your consultant, depending on how close they are to finishing their training. If you want to guarantee that your consultant will perform all of your operation, you may need to have surgery privately.

When will you meet your consultant surgeon?

You might meet your consultant when you are first assessed in the breast clinic. Alternatively, if you were seen by a nurse or junior doctor, you might meet your consultant when you get your results. Finally, some patients do not meet their consultant surgeon until the day of their operation.

Can you ask for a different surgeon?

Most patients feel confident with the surgeon looking after them. They have an open and trusting relationship with them and feel they can ask them anything, no matter how small or stupid it may seem. Occasionally, however, patients don't get on with their surgeon, normally because they don't like their bedside manner, and find that they are too direct. Sometimes patients can also feel that they are not being listened to.

If you aren't happy, you could ask your breast care nurse whether you could see a different consultant. Alternatively, you could ask your GP to refer you to another hospital, although this will delay your cancer treatment by a couple of weeks.

Are you fit enough to have an operation?

Before you can have your operation, your surgeon needs to make sure that you are fit enough to have an anaesthetic. Anaesthetics have several complications which can be serious (though these are rare – see page 126). Before your operation, you will be seen in a pre-assessment clinic by a doctor or a nurse to make sure that you can cope with the anaesthetic and the surgery. You may have a blood test, as well as a chest X-ray or a tracing of your heart rhythm (ECG).

The pre-assessment clinic will give you information about what to bring into hospital, where to go and when, whether you should take your normal medicines in the morning, and when to stop eating and drinking. If you are having a day-case operation you will need someone to take you home and stay with you overnight. If you live alone and have nobody to help you, you will probably be advised to stay in hospital for one night.

If you aren't fit enough to have a general anaesthetic (for example, you have serious heart, lung or kidney problems), your surgeon might be able to do your surgery using only local anaesthetic. This numbs your skin and tissues, so although you may feel pushing and pulling while your surgeon removes your cancer, it shouldn't hurt. You may also have a medicine to make you feel a little sleepy, so you won't really be aware of what is happening.

WHAT TO PACK FOR YOUR OPERATION

With many operations, patients go home on the same day, but you may stay longer, depending on what operation you are having. This checklist will help you pack:

ESSENTIALS

- Purse with a little money (hospitals aren't secure and things do get stolen).
- Mobile phone/tablet and charger.
- Books/magazines, etc. to keep you entertained.

TOILETRIES

- What you'd take for a weekend away – toothbrush and toothpaste as a bare minimum (hospital bathrooms just have hand soap).

CLOTHES

- Dressing gown to put over your hospital gown to keep you warm.
- A couple of spare pairs of knickers.
- Soft, non-wired bra for after the operation – front-fastening if you can find one (see page 109).
- Comfy clothes to go home in – ideally shirts and cardigans that you don't need to pull over your head.
- Sleepwear – pyjamas are easier than a nightdress for your doctor to examine you.
- Slippers or non-slip footwear.

MEDICATION

- All your normal tablets along with a written list of when you take them and what dose (the 'repeat prescription' printout from your GP is a good source of this).

The anaesthetic

Anaesthesia means 'without sensation'. There are two forms of anaesthetic – general and local. Most breast cancer operations are done using a general anaesthetic. This is a combination of drugs given by an anaesthetist (a doctor trained in giving anaesthetics) which make sure you are deeply asleep, unable to move and unable to feel pain during your operation (i.e. unconscious). Because an anaesthetic relaxes all your muscles, it means that the normal reflexes that stop food going into your windpipe don't work. If you were sick during the surgery, food could travel into your lungs and cause pneumonia. Therefore you need to have empty stomach when you have a general anaesthetic to stop this happening. Your surgeon will also use a local anaesthetic drug to numb the wound and reduce the pain afterwards.

One of the main side effects of anaesthetic is feeling sick or being sick. This doesn't happen to everyone, and you will be given medicine to prevent this. If you've been sick after an anaesthetic before, tell your anaesthetist. There is also a very small chance that you might be allergic to one of the drugs being used.

You might have a sore throat when you wake up because your anaesthetist will put a tube down your throat to help you breathe when you are asleep. If you have wobbly or loose teeth, there is also a risk that your teeth might be damaged or even fall out when the tube is put into your throat, though this is rare.

There are several complications that can happen with a general anaesthetic, and these include clots in the veins in your legs which can travel to your lungs, as well as heart and lung problems that can be very serious, especially if you have a relevant medical condition, such as emphysema or heart failure. These and other conditions might mean that the risks from a general anaesthetic are higher for you. Your nurse or doctor will talk to you about this when you go to the pre-assessment clinic.

THE DAY OF YOUR OPERATION
Arriving on the ward

You may be told to go to a main ward or to a waiting area next to the operating theatre. You will be taken to a bed where someone will get you ready for your operation, including giving you a hospital gown to put on and some compression socks to reduce the chance of getting a clot in your leg veins. If you are having simple breast surgery, you will be able to keep your own knickers on. If you are having a reconstruction involving your tummy, thighs or bottom, you will have to take your knickers off and may be given a sterile paper pair to put on. If you wear glasses, a wig or have dentures, you can keep these on/in until you are in the operating theatre. They should be at your bedside when you wake up.

Your anaesthetist will see you to explain what they are going to do, check your teeth and answer your questions. You will also meet either your consultant surgeon or one of their trainees who will check that you understand what operation you are going to have, answer any final questions, and mark your skin to show what side you are having surgery on (normally with a large arrow). They may also draw some additional guidelines to help guide them while you are asleep.

If someone has come with you to the hospital, they can wait with you while you are getting ready, but they can't go with you to the operating theatre. Some hospitals have a waiting room, but it might be nicer for your relative or friend to wait in a coffee shop, or even go home. One of the ward staff will call them when you are back on the ward.

Having your operation

You may either walk to theatre or be pushed in a wheelchair, bed or trolley, depending on where you are waiting. You will either have your anaesthetic in a small anteroom or in the operating theatre itself. After your operation, you will wake up in a special recovery area where there are nurses and doctors to monitor you. Your surgeon will come to see you, but you might not remember seeing them due to the effects of the anaesthetic. When you are properly awake (which can take up to an hour), you will be taken back to the ward to have something to eat and drink.

Most patients now go home on the same day. If you are staying in overnight, you should be seen by a doctor every day, but it might be someone you haven't met before, especially if you have your operation on a Friday.

Drains

A drain is a long plastic tube, stitched to your skin, which is connected to a bottle. It uses suction to drain any fluid that collects in your wound. Some surgeons use very small drains to infuse local anaesthetic into your wound; these are removed before you go home. If you have had a more complex breast operation or have had a lot of lymph nodes removed from your armpit, you may be sent home with your drains. In this case, you will be given detailed instructions about how to look after them. The tubing on a drain is deliberately long so you can (for example) put the drain bottle on the floor and stand up without it pulling. If you have a drain, you will probably be given a short course of antibiotics to reduce the chance of a wound infection. Your drain may be removed at home by a district nurse, or you may have it removed in the breast clinic. Drains typically stay in for 3–5 days.

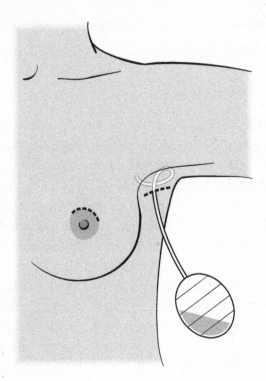

Drain after armpit surgery

Going home

You should see a breast care nurse before you go home. They will tell you how to look after your wounds, give you advice about wearing bras and staying active when you are at home. You will be shown some shoulder exercises (see page 229) and will be given an appointment to come back for your results. They will also make sure that you know who to call if you have a problem at home. If you've had a mastectomy, you might be given a heart-shaped mastectomy pillow to use under your arm when you go to sleep, and if you have a drain, you should also be given a bag to keep the drain in (you will need to give it back when you next see your surgeon). Drain bags and mastectomy pillows can also be bought online.

> Trish woke up from her mastectomy attached to various monitors recording her pulse, blood oxygen level and blood pressure. She wasn't in any pain, but she felt a bit sick. She vomited once and felt much better. Her surgeon came to see her, but she doesn't remember it. An hour after returning to the ward, she had a sandwich and a cup of tea. The next morning, the nurses removed her drain and let her go home. She was well enough to go out for a meal with her family that same evening.
>
> Liz can't remember being in recovery at all, and only remembers waking up on the ward. However, her lovely husband videoed Liz declaring her undying love for him under the influence of morphine. She didn't believe it until she saw the video. She had very little pain and went home the next day with her drains still in place.

RECOVERING FROM YOUR OPERATION

You will probably be a little sore after your operation. It is normally your armpit wound that hurts the most because you move your arms all the time, whereas your breast just sits in a bra. You will hopefully have been advised to buy some simple painkillers to take at home, and it is important to take them regularly. You can have 1g of paracetamol up to four times a day, and 400mg of ibuprofen (if it's safe for you to take it) up to three times a day. Keeping active after your surgery (gentle walking) and doing your shoulder exercises will also help ease the pain. If you have had a large operation, like a reconstruction, it will be more painful. In this case, your doctor will prescribe some stronger painkillers, such as liquid morphine, to take as well.

When will you get back to normal?

After your operation, you will need to spend a minimum of one to two weeks recovering at home. If you are working, you can write yourself a sick note for the first week, but your surgeon or GP will need to give you one for the rest of your time away from work. If you have had a reconstruction (see Chapter 8), you might need several months off.

Take it easy for the first few days, but don't spend hours on end lying on the sofa as this can increase the risk of you developing a blood clot in your leg. You should be able to do basic activities like getting washed and dressed without too much discomfort, and you should aim to walk regularly. It isn't safe to drive until you can safely do an emergency stop without pausing to think whether it might hurt, and can easily turn to look behind you when reversing. This normally takes two weeks, so you might need to plan ahead and get help with things like food shopping and school runs. It is normal to feel tired after an operation, and you may feel that you need an afternoon nap for the first week or two until your energy levels pick up. You may also still be dealing with the emotional aftermath of a breast cancer diagnosis, so be kind to yourself and don't stress too much if the laundry isn't done and the house isn't spotless.

You should see your doctor after two weeks to have your wound checked. If you have had a reduction or a reconstruction, you may have your wound looked at after a week. If your wound has healed and your surgeon is happy, they will give you the okay to go back to work and to exercise properly. They will also tell you when you can start wearing an underwired bra again.

Your doctor will also give you your results and discuss with you what other treatments you might need. The one treatment that most people are scared of is chemotherapy, and we both needed it. In the next chapter, we're going to explain what chemotherapy is, what happens when you have it and, more importantly, tell you all our tips to help you cope with the symptoms.

CHAPTER 10

CHEMOTHERAPY

CHEMOTHERAPY (OR 'CHEMO') is a cancer treatment used to kill cancer cells, although healthy cells are also affected. The drugs damage cells and stop them growing. Normal cells can usually repair the damage, but cancer cells can't and so they die.

When do you have chemotherapy?

Most patients have chemotherapy after their surgery but before radiotherapy. This is called 'adjuvant chemotherapy'.

You may be advised to have chemotherapy before surgery, particularly if you are young, have positive nodes or have inflammatory breast cancer (see page 14). Chemotherapy is also used to try and shrink a large cancer so you don't need a mastectomy, and sometimes the breast cancer completely disappears. This is called 'neoadjuvant chemotherapy'. It is more effective in women with triple negative cancers. If your cancer is HER2-positive, having neoadjuvant chemotherapy means you can have an additional drug called Perjeta that also targets HER2 and can improve your prognosis (see Chapter 11). It can also buy you time to get the results from a BRCA test (see page 3) which could affect your surgical decisions.

Is chemotherapy worth the risk?

If you have primary breast cancer, surgery gives you the greatest chance of a cure. Chemotherapy is used to reduce the risk of a recurrence. We discussed how doctors determine whether you will benefit from chemotherapy in Chapter 3 (page 31). Before recommending chemotherapy, your oncologist will also consider your general health and lifestyle. Chemotherapy can be gruelling, even for the youngest, fittest patients. It is offered to older patients, but your doctor needs to make sure that you're fit enough to cope with it, and that the benefits outweigh the risks.

Some cancer patients refuse chemotherapy for a variety of reasons. The most common reason is not wanting to lose their hair (although there are now cold caps to help you keep it – see page 142) or wanting to try alternative therapies instead. Please remember, if your doctors are recommending chemotherapy, it means that your risk of the cancer coming back is already high and, at the moment, there aren't any other comparable treatments that have been proven to reduce this risk.

How long does chemotherapy take?

If you have primary breast cancer, your chemotherapy will normally take between three and five months. It is given in 'cycles', a cycle being the time between each treatment. Each cycle can be one, two or three weeks long, depending on which drugs you are having. The cycles give your body time to recover and repair the healthy cells that were damaged, and let you recover from the side effects before the next cycle starts.

If you have secondary breast cancer, you may be recommended to have treatment for the rest of your life. Which drugs you have will depend on the extent of your disease and where in your body it is. Breast cancers can become resistant to chemotherapy drugs, so you might have to switch from one drug to another to keep the cancer under control.

How will your health be monitored during chemotherapy?

You will have blood taken before each cycle to make sure that your immune system is strong enough to cope with chemotherapy. The test measures the number of neutrophils (a type of white blood cell) in your blood. Because chemotherapy affects your bone marrow (where blood cells are made), the number of neutrophils in your blood tends to fall with every cycle. If you don't have enough neutrophils, your chemotherapy will be postponed until your blood test reaches a threshold level where it is safe to give you another dose. The blood test will also check that your liver and kidneys are working well enough to withstand the next dose.

If you have neoadjuvant chemotherapy, you may have a breast MRI to monitor the response of your cancer to chemotherapy. If the MRI indicates that your cancer is growing, your oncologist will stop treatment, ask your surgeon to operate, and then continue chemotherapy once you've recovered from the surgery.

Your oncologist will see you regularly to ask you about the side effects you may have had and answer any questions. They will examine you, review your blood tests and scans and prescribe drugs to help with the side effects and any other drugs you need to take at home.

QUESTIONS TO ASK YOUR
ONCOLOGIST/SPECIALIST ONCOLOGY NURSE

- Why are you recommending chemotherapy?
- What happens if I don't have it?
- How will you know if it's working?
- What happens if it doesn't work?
- Where will I have chemotherapy?
- How long does it take?
- What are the side effects, when will they happen and how long will they last?
- Are there research trials I could go on to?
- Is there anything I should and shouldn't do during treatment?
- How long does it take for the side effects to start?
- What do I need to monitor at home?
- What do I do if I feel unwell at home during the day, in the evenings and at weekends?

CHEMOTHERAPY DRUGS

There are several different chemotherapy drugs that are used in different combinations. Your oncologist will decide which is best for you based on the specific details of your breast cancer and the results from years of research trials.

You will get detailed information about each of the drugs you have, and that information can also be found on, and downloaded from, the Macmillan, Breast Cancer Care and Cancer Research UK websites (see pages 277–80 for details). Most chemotherapy drugs are given with other medicines, like antihistamines and steroids, to stop you getting an allergic reaction, and to help with sickness and vomiting.

Chemotherapy for primary breast cancer

These are the some of the common drugs that are used:

- FEC (Fluorouracil (5FU), Epirubicin and Cyclophosphamide)
- FEC-T (FEC then a Taxane – Docetaxel (Taxotere) or Paclitaxol (Taxol))
- T-FEC (Taxane then FEC)
- AC or EC (Doxorubicin (Adriamycin) or Epirubicin and Cyclophosphamide)
- Platinum-based (Carboplatin and Cisplatin)
- CMF (Cyclophosphamide, Methotrexate and 5FU)

Most chemotherapy regimens now include a taxane (third-generation chemotherapy). If you have a BRCA mutation or a triple negative cancer you will probably get a platinum-based agent.

Chemotherapy for secondary breast cancer

These are some of the chemo drugs used for secondary cancer, but they may only be available as part of a research trial:

- AC (see above)
- Capecitabine (Xeloda)
- Carboplatin
- Cisplatin
- Eribulin (Halaven)
- Gemcitabine (Gemvar)
- Vinorelbine (Navelbine)

Additional targeted therapies for secondary cancer such as CDK4/6 inhibitors (immunotherapy) are discussed in Chapter 11.

HAVING CHEMOTHERAPY

Most drugs are given into a vein (intravenously), but some come as tablets. There are three ways to give chemo intravenously:

Cannula

A cannula is a short plastic tube put into a vein, normally on the back of your hand. It is removed after each treatment. Chemotherapy drugs can irritate and scar your veins which can make it harder to find a good vein each time.

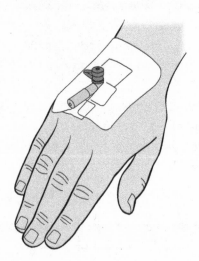

Cannula

PICC line (peripherally inserted central catheter)

This is a much longer cannula which is put into a vein in your arm, just above your elbow, and ends in a large vein that goes to your heart. It's put in using local anaesthetic and stays in place until you have finished chemotherapy. You can also have blood taken through it. It's covered with a waterproof dressing which needs to be changed every week. You can buy coloured PICC line covers from websites such as Live Better With Cancer: https://livebetterwith.com

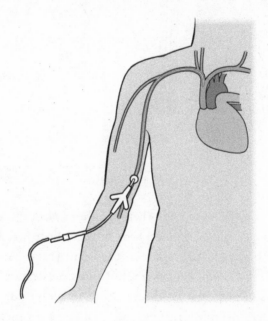

PICC line

Port

A long cannula is put into a large central vein in your chest. It's connected to a 'port' which sits just under your skin, normally below your collarbone. The drugs are given through the port which is punctured using a needle, and trained nurses can also take blood from it. It is normally put in using local anaesthetic and sedation and stays in until you have finished chemotherapy.

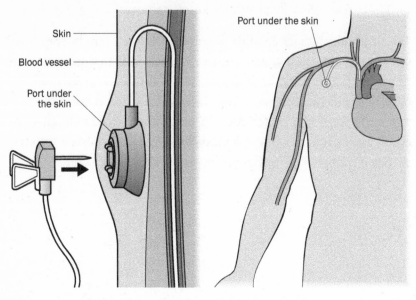

Skin

Blood vessel

Port under the skin

Port under the skin

Port

Where do you have chemotherapy?

Most patients will have chemotherapy in an oncology day unit in a hospital. You should be given a tour of the unit before you start. If not, ask for one as it makes it less scary on the day. Also ask what food and drink is available, as a lot of units provide only tap water (you can take your own food and drink in with you). Most units have large, comfortable reclining chairs for you to sit in, and if you're going privately you'll probably be shown directly to your own cubicle. Alternatively, you may sit on a trolley. There will probably be other patients sat in the chairs next to you. Some hospitals now have mobile chemo units, which means that if you live a long distance from the hospital, the chemo van may come to a place near you. A few large primary care centres (GP practices) can also give chemotherapy.

What should you wear?

You can wear whatever you like! You need to be comfortable as you may be there for several hours. If you have a port or a PICC (see pages 137 and 138), your nurse needs to be able to access it, so wear a short-sleeved top, and no polo necks. You may want to dress up and make an occasion out of it, especially for your last cycle, so feel free to get inspired.

What actually happens?

Once your blood results have come back (if you have them on the day of chemo), and there is a free chair for you to sit in, you will meet a chemotherapy nurse who will give you your drugs. In our experience, chemo nurses are fantastic at making you feel as relaxed as possible. They also know about the side effects of the drugs you're being given and how scary it feels, so talk to them. Some drugs are left to infuse into your veins over an hour, while others (like FEC) have to be injected slowly by hand, which means the nurse will sit with you for one to two hours while they administer them. Having chemo can be lonely, especially if everyone around you has visitors. It's nice if you can find a relative or friend to come and sit with you. On the other hand, you might just want to get lost in a book or a film/box set.

How long does it take?

The time varies depending on which drugs you are having, and how they are being given. It normally takes one to two hours. If you are using a cold cap, you may be in the chemo unit for up to six hours (see page 142).

Travelling to and from chemotherapy

Most people feel well enough to make their own way to the hospital, either by driving or using public transport. However, after you have had chemo you may not feel well enough to drive yourself home. Sometimes the side effects kick in quickly, and you may feel sick or tired on the bus or Tube home. We advise getting someone to take you home each time if you can, especially if you have some distance to travel.

WHAT SHOULD YOU TAKE?

This is what we took with us:

- Entertainment – books, magazines, crosswords, headphones to listen to music, a tablet loaded with box sets or films
- Phone and a charger
- Food and drink – water can taste awful, so taking squash to flavour it can help
- Warm socks and slippers or flip-flops so you don't slip when going to the toilet
- Gloves, a scarf and a warm blanket if you are cold-capping (see page 142)

How will your body react?

It normally takes 12–24 hours for the effects to kick in, and often starts with a funny taste in your mouth followed by flu or hangover symptoms which get worse over the next couple of days. This slowly improves over the next few days until you feel almost normal. Everyone has a different pattern, and you will come to learn which are your really bad days. As the cycles progress, you will find that you don't bounce back as quickly or as high as you did in the beginning, since the drugs gradually accumulate in your body. However, you will still get your good days and weeks, and it's worth bearing in mind that, as you get more tired, you're nearing the end of your treatment.

SIDE EFFECTS AND COMPLICATIONS

Because chemotherapy targets any cells that are rapidly dividing, this means that your hair, skin, nails, taste buds, the lining of your gut, and your bone marrow (which produces blood cells) are all affected and this explains the various side effects. Most of these side effects disappear when you finish chemo, although you may be left with some 'collateral damage' – long-term side effects that might not improve, such as numbness in your fingers and toes, called 'peripheral neuropathy' (see page 150). It can take six to twelve months to fully recover. Some studies suggest that chemotherapy can biologically 'age' you by up to 10 years, though this will depend on which drugs you receive and how you react to them.

Before we start talking about the side effects, here are the two most important lessons we learned to minimise your body's reaction to the drugs:

1. Drink 2–3 litres of water every day. It helps flush out the chemotherapy, it rehydrates you and you *will* feel better for it.
2. Walk for 30 minutes *every* day. Try to do this even when you feel ghastly; even when you have to stop to catch your breath, spit or be sick every 10 minutes; even when you can only walk to the end of the road and back because you're so out of breath. Lots of studies have shown that regular exercise reduces the side effects of chemotherapy, and we both saw the benefits from daily exercise. Try to persuade someone to walk with you. You'll hate us for making you do it, but it will make you feel better. We promise. If you're an athlete, we cover training and exercise during chemotherapy in Chapter 18.

Losing your hair

The most common side effect of chemotherapy is hair loss and it's the one that most people are afraid of. You lose *all* your hair – pubic, leg, chest, underarm, facial hair, and, towards the end of your treatment, your eyebrows and eyelashes (because they grow more slowly). Hair loss normally starts at around Day 13. Your pubic hair often falls out first, followed by clumps of hair that collect on your hairbrush or the bottom of the shower.

Even though Liz knew this was going to happen, she still cried in the shower when her first clump of hair came out. Being bald can be very hard to cope with, especially if your hair is an important part of your image. Losing your hair can stop you feeling feminine and make you very self-conscious when you leave the house. There are lots of ways to cope with being bald, which we'll cover below, and you can even have fun with it. But first, let's talk about cold-capping, which is something you can do to try and keep the hair on your head, like Trish.

Cold-capping

This is a tight rubber cap with freezing cold fluid running through it, covered with a neoprene hat with a chin strap to keep it in place. The freezing temperature lowers the blood flow to your scalp and reduces the effect of the drugs on your hair. It works in around half the people who try it, and it worked for Trish. (She had short hair to start with, and only had a bit of thinning, although she still lost her eyebrows, eyelashes and pubic hair.)

The cap has to fit tightly to work, especially at the top of your head where hair loss would be most obvious. Be fussy and make sure it fits properly. You wear the cap for half an hour before and up to one hour after each infusion. You will feel cold, and you might get an 'ice cream headache', so wear warm gloves, scarves and socks, and you could also take a heated electric blanket. It's a good idea to take some paracetamol beforehand.

You must be really gentle with your hair. If it is very long, you might want to cut it to shoulder length so it's easier to manage. Wash it no more than once or twice a week with a gentle shampoo; take care when brushing (use a wide-toothed brush or comb and hold your hair at the roots) and avoid heat (such as hairdryers and straighteners).

Braving the shave

When your hair does start to fall out, you might want to shave it off in one go rather than deal with the mess (and emotional fall-out) of losing it over a few days or weeks and having a very straggly, thinning, head of hair. The shave is never going to be easy. Some people make an occasion of it and throw a party or open a bottle of bubbly and get their partner to do it. If this isn't something that appeals, you can ask your hairdresser to do it, like Liz did. However you do it, you will almost certainly cry. Most hairdressers can squeeze you in on the day (as it's hard to predict when you need to do it) and they normally don't charge you.

There are many options for covering your head. Synthetic wigs are available on the NHS, but you may have to pay some of the cost. Human hair wigs are more realistic, but also more expensive. You may find a shorter hairstyle is more practical or choose a longer wig and cut it short as your hair starts to grow again. Wigs can be very hot to wear, especially if you have hot flushes, and you may find you don't wear yours around the house.

Many people prefer to wear a scarf or hat instead. There are lots of websites selling headwear for cancer patients, ranging from simple cotton beanies to showy turbans for special occasions. Macmillan and Breast Cancer Care have a good list of retailers on their websites (see 178 and 181 for details). Tying headscarves is an art in itself – you can find videos on YouTube. If you do buy a hat, it might be too big for you without your hair, but you can buy hat adjuster pads that stick inside the brim to make them fit.

You may decide to be 'bald and proud', like Liz. It is scary going out in public for the first time (you'll think everyone is looking at you and talking about you) but it gets easier. You can have fun with temporary tattoos and henna crowns, or even have a Turkish shave in a men's barber shop. If you want to shave your head to keep it smooth, use a fresh blade every time, and get someone to help you do the parts you can't see.

Eyelashes and eyebrows

Losing your eyelashes and eyebrows can be even harder to cope with as they help define your face. You might want to get your eyebrows 'micro-bladed' (semi-permanent make-up) before you start treatment. The free 'Look Good Feel Better' course (see page 184) will teach you how to draw on eyebrows, and there are lots of videos online. A fine eyeliner can help mimic eyelashes. False lashes are hard to stick on when you don't have any of your own and should be avoided if your skin is sensitive or sore. Your brows and lashes normally grow back within 2–3 months. There are expensive serums available that claim to speed up regrowth, but we're not aware of the evidence behind them. We didn't use them, and our lashes and brows grew back a few weeks after we finished chemo.

Managing your new hair

Your hair should start to grow back a couple of weeks after your last cycle, with a full head of hair within six months. When your hair does grow back, it may be a different colour and texture from your original hair, and often it first grows back as grey 'chemo curls'. No one really knows why this happens. If you are young, your hair may return to your normal colour and texture, but if your hair had already started to go grey, it may remain grey and curly.

Your new hair will be fragile, like baby hair, and you don't want to damage it, so wait at least six months before colouring it. Ideally get your hairdresser to do this for you, but if you can't wait that long, use vegetable-based and henna dyes, and avoid anything permanent.

Serious infection (neutropenic sepsis)

Because chemotherapy reduces the number of white blood cells (neutrophils) needed to fight infection, you're more likely to get an infection during chemo which could potentially become life-threatening within a few hours if it isn't treated. This is called 'neutropenic sepsis'. It happened to both of us.

Your neutrophils start to drop halfway through each cycle and should return to normal in time for your next treatment. You may be given a course of antibiotics to reduce the risk of infection and your oncologist may also prescribe a drug called G-CSF. This stimulates your bone marrow to make more white blood cells. G-CSF is given as a daily or weekly injection (you can learn to give it yourself into the skin of your tummy or thigh). It can sting a little and does have significant side effects (bone pain, headaches, fever and flu-like symptoms), but it's worth it to reduce the risk of you getting an infection.

When to suspect a serious infection

The earliest warning sign of neutropenic sepsis is usually a rise in your temperature. You'll be told to check your temperature twice a day. It is worth spending money on an accurate digital thermometer that goes in your ear because the cheaper models you put under your tongue can break and give faulty readings. You'll be given a 24-hour emergency contact number, and you should call it if you have any of the following symptoms:

- your temperature is above 37.5°C or 38°C (depending on the advice you've been given)
- you suddenly feel unwell, even with a normal temperature
- you feel shivery and can't stop shaking
- you have symptoms of an infection such as a cold, sore throat, cough, passing urine frequently or diarrhoea

You need to take these symptoms seriously, as any infection could be life-threatening. When you call the hospital, you will be told to either go straight to the oncology unit or to the A&E department. Unless you are very poorly, you don't need to call for an ambulance, but you should leave the house within 15–20 minutes.

It's a good idea to have an overnight bag packed ready to go, with a toothbrush, toothpaste and mouthwash, hand cream and lip salve, Vaseline, phone charger, notebook and pen, pyjamas, socks and slippers, a nice pillowcase (hospital ones aren't soft), a list of the tablets you're taking, something to entertain you, squash or flavoured water and snacks that you can eat (hospital food isn't always the best thing to eat when you feel sick and everything tastes funny).

> Liz was told she needed to pack a bag but didn't because she never thought she would get a serious infection. When her temperature did rise and she had to go into hospital, she felt so awful it was hard to concentrate on what to pack.

What happens when you go to hospital with a suspected infection?

You need to be quickly assessed by a doctor or nurse and given antibiotics into a vein within 60 minutes of being seen, usually before any blood tests or scan results come back. It is vital that you get these antibiotics promptly. Make sure you tell the person seeing you that you are having chemotherapy, so they know how important it is to give you the antibiotics quickly.

If your blood tests confirm that you have an infection you will be kept in hospital for a day or two (occasionally longer) to have more antibiotics through a cannula, before being sent home with antibiotic tablets. Often the blood results are normal and the high temperature was a false alarm, but it is better to be safe than sorry.

HOW TO REDUCE YOUR INFECTION RISK

- Stay away from anyone with a cough or cold, tummy bug or chickenpox.
- Avoid places like Jacuzzis, and public transport in the rush hour, especially in winter.
- If you have pets, always wash your hands after touching them, and wear gloves when cleaning up after them.

- Make sure you wash your hands before you eat and after you've been to the toilet.
- Clean your bottom gently but thoroughly after opening your bowels, and always wipe front to back.
- Brush your teeth and use a mouthwash after every meal.
- Use moisturiser and hand cream to stop your skin cracking.
- Use gloves when gardening and washing up, and don't trim the cuticles of your nails.
- Use a fresh blade every time you shave or use an electric shaver.

Foods to avoid when your immunity is low

You are at risk of getting an infection from contaminated food. You should avoid food that is out of date, in damaged packaging or loose (such as bread rolls, salad from salad bars, food from deli counters and 'pick'n'mix' sweets that other people may have touched).

Some other tips to avoid infection include:

- Buy vacuum-packed meat and cheese.
- Avoid raw and rare meat, raw fish, shellfish and blue cheese.
- Cook eggs until the yolks are firm.
- Keep and prepare raw meat and vegetables separately.
- Wash and peel all raw fruit and vegetables.
- Always wash your hands after preparing food.

Food, taste and smell

Chemotherapy alters your sense of taste and smell. You will have a funny taste in your mouth (often chalky or metallic) and things you normally love to eat and drink may taste awful. It can be hard to find things you do want to eat and drink. Although your taste may come back a little before each cycle, things never taste quite the same until after you've stopped treatment.

Working out what to eat can be very hard. There are several cookbooks available to help. Our favourite was *The Royal Marsden Cancer Cookbook* edited by cancer dietician Dr Clare Shaw (Kyle Books, 2015). It tells you what to try for different tastes, what to eat when it's painful to swallow and what to eat if you need to gain or lose weight. Many recipes can be cooked in bulk and frozen in your good weeks.

If your mouth is very sore, stick to soft foods such as ice cream, smoothies, yoghurt and mashed potato. Try using strong flavourings (e.g. chilli, soy sauce) so you can actually taste something. Pineapple can help when things taste chalky and your tongue is coated. Experiment with new combinations and if you find something that works, stick with it. Liz survived on soggy Weetabix and maple syrup for breakfast because even sugar grains were too scratchy on her mouth. Trish had cheese on toast (with the crusts cut off) for supper every day for three months. If you've really lost your appetite or are very nauseous, set a reminder on your phone every couple of hours (or ask someone to prompt you) and try to get something down. Finally, it's okay to drink alcohol and eat chocolate on your good days. Enjoy your taste buds while they're recovering.

Although we recommended that you drink 2–3 litres of water a day, chemo gives it a horrible taste. Use lemons or cordial to flavour it and get used to carrying a bottle around with you and refill it at every meal time. Tonic water can also help to cut through the chalky taste in your mouth. You may find tea and coffee taste differently too, so if you want a hot drink, try hot squash or adding Bovril, Marmite or Vegemite to hot water.

Other side effects
Head and face

Headaches are common and these normally respond to paracetamol, though occasionally you may need a stronger painkiller like codeine. You may get red flushed cheeks and acne on your face, and steroids can make your face look swollen. You can also get a painful spot on the edge of your eyelid called a stye. Use a hot compress to reduce the swelling and see your GP if it doesn't settle.

Nose and mouth

The lining of your nose can get sore and bleed because you lose your protective nose hairs. Smear some Vaseline inside your nostrils to keep them moist. Your lips will get dry and can crack and split, so make sure you use a thick lip balm (such as Lanolips) regularly. The inside of your mouth can become sore and you may get ulcers on your tongue and gums. Your GP can prescribe an oral gel (such as Gelclair) that coats the ulcers and eases the pain. Your gums can bleed, and you might find it painful to swallow. Use a soft baby toothbrush after every meal with a gentle toothpaste like Biotene. Then rinse your mouth with a gentle medicated mouthwash such as Difflam, which your GP can prescribe.

Digestive system

You can get indigestion which your GP can treat with a tablet or a medicine. Most people feel sick, and you may vomit. Your oncologist will prescribe you an anti-sickness tablet (such as Ondansetron, Cyclizine or Emend). If one tablet doesn't work, tell your doctor and they can try another – don't suffer in silence. Lemon and ginger tea, sweets and biscuits can also help with nausea, and some people use magnetic wrist bands to ease the sickness.

Your bowel habits will change, and you will either have frequent watery stools (diarrhoea) or not go for days at a time (constipation). When you do eventually go, it may be painful and cause haemorrhoids (piles). Try changing your diet and adding more fruit and fibre (such as figs and prunes which are natural laxatives), if you can stand the taste of them. You will probably also need a variety of medicines and tablets to help as well, which your oncologist or GP can prescribe for you.

Hands and feet

Your nails will soften, crack, split, or even fall off, and you may get brown spots underneath them. A nail-strengthening polish can help stop your nails feeling sore. Some people develop 'hand-foot syndrome' which causes a tightness, burning or redness in the skin of your hands and feet, peeling, cracked skin, blisters, ulcers and difficulty walking or using your hands. Use a thick hand cream regularly to keep your skin soft, wear gloves when washing up, use gentle, moisturising hand soap and don't spend a long time soaking in hot water. Wear sensible, well-fitting shoes.

Chemotherapy can also damage the nerves in your fingers and toes (called 'peripheral neuropathy') which reduces your ability to feel pain and changes in temperature and makes it difficult to do fiddly tasks such as doing up buttons. These symptoms normally improve but they can be permanent. If you are affected, your oncologist may need to reduce your chemotherapy dose.

Joints and muscles

You might have generalised aches and pains, notice that your arms and legs swell, or get cramps. Regular painkillers will help with the aches and pains. Sit or lie with your legs raised on a cushion to help the swelling go down.

'Chemo brain'

You will probably find it hard to concentrate on anything in the first few days of chemo, and this is called 'chemo brain'. It can feel like you are living in a foggy cloud, and you literally can't focus on a book or the TV for more than a few minutes at a time. You might struggle to find the right words or to remember simple things. It normally gets better as each day passes, so ride it out. It might help to keep a notepad close to hand to write down important things. Liz did jigsaws because she could dip in and out for a few minutes at a time and feel she'd accomplished something. Some people are still affected months and even years later. Liz still gets words muddled up from time to time, and that's three years after treatment. Doing puzzles and brain-training games can help, as well as yoga and mindfulness techniques (see Chapters 14 and 18 for more on this).

Fatigue

Chemotherapy drugs and the medication given to reduce side effects can make you fatigued. Fatigue means mental and physical exhaustion that doesn't get better after resting. We cover this in more detail in Chapter 15 (page 193).

Insomnia

If you are given steroids to help with the side effects, they can cause insomnia for a couple of days. This means that you can't get to sleep and lie awake all night, which can be exacerbated if you're in a lot of pain or are worrying. Make sure you've taken your painkillers. If you can't get back to sleep, don't fight it. Watch a TV show, read a magazine or chat to friends on forums (someone is always awake at 3am!).

Menopause

Chemotherapy can affect your ovaries and bring on an instant menopause. See Chapter 16 for advice on symptom control and fertility preservation.

Effects on diabetes

If you have diabetes, the combination of irregular and unusual meals along with steroids can make your diabetes unstable, with your blood sugar either too high or too low. If you take insulin, you will need to check your blood sugar level more regularly during treatment. Your oncologist may need to liaise with your diabetes specialist, your GP and/or a dietician to ensure that you have a workable plan for getting through chemo.

HOW TO COPE WITH CHEMOTHERAPY

There is no magic formula for getting through chemo, but here are some of the things that worked for us. We hope they will help you too.

Getting through the bad days

Make a 'chemo caddy' – a little box or bag that you keep next to you when you are lying on the sofa. It should have lip balm, hand cream, your thermometer, painkillers, a small notebook and pen, and a magazine or two. Invest in a warm, fleecy blanket to snuggle under. You might want to keep a duplicate set of toothbrush/toothpaste/mouthwash in a downstairs bathroom so you can brush your teeth after eating when you don't have the energy to climb the stairs.

Self-monitoring

You need to take your temperature regularly, monitor your side effects and look out for signs of an infection. Keep a notepad close by to write down symptoms as they happen, because chemo brain can make it hard to remember things. You might also want to record your pulse rate, energy levels, exercise, sleep and bowel movements, and most smartphones have health apps that you can use to do this.

The free Macmillan 'My Organiser' app is a great resource (search for it on the Apple App Store or Google Play). It will set up reminders on your phone telling you when to take your tablets and drugs, as well as your appointments for blood tests and hospital visits. It also has links to the side effects of the drugs you're taking as well as somewhere to store your emergency contact numbers.

You won't feel great during chemotherapy but you're not meant to feel really terrible, though it's hard to know what is the normal level of suffering when you're having it for the first time. Don't suffer in silence. If in doubt, call your oncology nurse and ask them for advice. Remember – you're never alone.

Life goes on

It's so important not to put your entire life on hold during chemo. How much you can work, play and join in family life will depend partly on how often you have your infusions, which drugs you're on and what your responsibilities are. You will soon work out the pattern of your bad and good days or weeks. When you feel well enough, meet up with friends, have a massage or go away for the weekend. If you have a special occasion like a wedding to go to, your doctor might be able to rearrange your chemo day so you're well enough to go.

And what about sex? Everyone feels differently about sex during chemotherapy. You may find that it's the last thing on your mind, but intimacy and sex can be a good way of connecting with your partner when everything around you feels like it's falling apart. See Chapter 17 for advice on relationships, sex and contraception.

Children, elderly relatives and pets are a fact of life. Ask family and friends to help with school runs, washing and ironing, walking the dogs, etc. If your house isn't spotless and your family eats take-away meals when you're feeling rough, who cares? It can be equally difficult if you live alone and there's no one to help look after you. Online forums and social media can help connect you with other people. It may also be worth asking someone to stay with you during your chemo 'bad days'.

No matter how bad you feel on your very worst days, you *will* get through chemotherapy, and we promise you that in a year from now, you won't remember how bad you felt. Liz wouldn't have believed you if you had told her this at the time, especially on her really bad days, but honestly, one year later she couldn't remember what it was like or how she felt. It's only when she gets a really bad cold that she remembers the days spent curled up on the sofa feeling miserable.

If you have secondary breast cancer and chemo is for life, you may need to have hard conversations with your oncologist about the trade-off between the side effects of chemo and the risk of delaying it for a treatment break, or stopping it altogether. We discuss this in more detail in Chapter 23.

Reading this chapter won't have been easy, and nobody wants to have chemotherapy. However, we hope that we've been able to throw you a lifeline and help you get through chemo if you need it.

CHAPTER 11

HERCEPTIN AND OTHER TARGETED THERAPIES

THIS CHAPTER COVERS targeted therapies used to treat HER2-positive breast cancers. But what does 'HER2-positive' actually mean? Every breast cancer cell produces a protein called Human Epidermal Growth Factor Receptor 2, called 'HER2'. HER2-positive cancers express very high levels of HER2, and 15–20 per cent of all breast cancers are HER2-positive (HER2+ve). The extra HER2 protein stimulates the cells to divide and grow much faster than HER2-negative (HER2-ve) cancers.

Years ago, HER2-positive cancers had a poor prognosis, but this was before the introduction of drugs like Herceptin. In 2012, a big review of research trials by the Cochrane Collaboration involving almost 12,000 women showed that Herceptin prevents one-third of breast cancer deaths in HER2-positive patients.

How do you know if your cancer is HER2-positive?

If your core biopsy (see page 25) shows an invasive cancer, it is first tested for HER2 positivity using a method called 'immuno-histochemistry'. This gives a score of 0, 1, 2 or 3. A score of 0 or 1 means that your cancer is HER2-negative. A score of 3 means that your cancer is HER2-positive. A score of 2 is a borderline result, and another test called 'In Situ Hybridisation' (FISH or CISH) is then done to confirm whether your cancer is HER2-positive or negative. Liz's cancer was HER2-negative, while Trish's was HER2-positive.

DRUGS FOR HER2-POSITIVE CANCERS

HER2-positive cancers are treated with drugs that specifically target the HER2 receptor on the outside of the breast cancer cell.

Herceptin

Herceptin (trastuzumab) is used to treat primary and secondary breast cancer. It is a monoclonal antibody (in other words, a large protein) that locks on to the HER2 protein and stops it working, which then stops the cancer cell from dividing and growing. Herceptin also helps the immune system attack and destroy breast cancer cells.

Perjeta

Perjeta (pertuzumab) is another monoclonal antibody that locks on to a different part of the HER2 protein. If you are having neo-adjuvant chemotherapy you may be given Perjeta and Herceptin (a combination known as 'dual anti-HER2 therapy'). Perjeta is also used to treat patients with secondary HER2-positive cancers.

Tyverb

Tyverb (lapatinib) locks on to the HER2 receptor and another epidermal growth factor receptor called HER1. It is currently only used to treat secondary HER2-positive breast cancer.

Kadcyla

Kadcyla (trastuzumab emtansine) is a combination of two drugs. The first, trastuzumab (Herceptin) locks onto the HER2 receptor. This then allows targeted delivery of the second drug, emtansine, directly into cancer cells which destroys them. Normal cells are unharmed so there are fewer side effects than with chemotherapy. Kadcyla is currently only used to treat secondary HER2-positive breast cancer.

Herceptin, Perjeta and Kadcyla are given by injections – either into your vein or under your skin. Most patients have them as an out-patient in hospital (often on the chemo unit), but they may be given in your GP surgery or at home. Tyverb comes as a tablet that you take every day.

WHEN AND HOW IS HER2 TREATMENT GIVEN?

At the time of writing, Herceptin can only be given with a course of chemotherapy. This is because all the evidence showing the benefit of Herceptin comes from research trials where patients were given both chemotherapy and Herceptin at the same time. This means that even if you have a very small HER2-positive cancer that hasn't spread to your lymph nodes, like Trish, you still need to have chemotherapy in order to get Herceptin treatment. Your oncologist may give you a gentler chemotherapy regime that is easier to tolerate, together with Herceptin, like Trish had. She was told to think of chemotherapy as a general poison that would make the cancer cells more susceptible to the 'silver bullet' of Herceptin.

Primary breast cancer

Herceptin is currently given once every three weeks for a total of 18 doses, which takes a year. If you have neoadjuvant chemotherapy, you'll have either Herceptin, or Herceptin and Perjeta (dual anti-HER2 therapy) at the same time. Once you've had surgery, you'll continue with Herceptin alone.

Secondary breast cancer

You may have Herceptin, Herceptin and Perjeta, or Tyverb together with chemotherapy. Your oncologist will determine which drugs you need based on your tumour type and spread, and its response to previous treatment.

Why you might not get HER2 treatment even if your cancer is HER2-positive

Herceptin cannot be given if you are pregnant or breastfeeding because it can damage your baby. You must use contraception during treatment and for at least six months after the date of your last Herceptin dose. If you have heart problems, you may not be able to have Herceptin because it can affect your heart (see page 159 for more on this).

How are the injections given?

The first injection is slow, and can take 90 minutes to give. It is normally given in to a vein (via a cannula, PICC or port) at the same time as your chemotherapy infusion. You are given anti-allergy drugs (such as steroids) to take first to reduce the risk of an allergic reaction, and you have to stay in the hospital for several hours to make sure that you feel okay afterwards. If it's given before chemo, the waiting time may have finished by the time your chemo drugs have been infused. The next injections are much shorter, and only take 30 minutes or so.

After your first dose, or once you have finished chemo, you can have your remaining treatments as an injection under the skin of your thigh, swapping sides each time. The first injection under the skin will be in the hospital and takes 3–5 minutes. You may then be able to have the remainder of your injections closer to home, instead of having to travel to the hospital.

Trish had Herceptin injected under the skin of her thigh. It didn't really hurt, apart from the initial prick when the needle went in. Sometimes she gave the injection herself at home.

SIDE EFFECTS AND COMPLICATIONS

Most people tolerate Herceptin very well and side effects are relatively rare. You may feel like you have a mild dose of the flu for a day or two after the treatment (aching muscles, a sore throat, sickness, loss of appetite, diarrhoea and exhaustion), but this normally eases with paracetamol.

> Trish didn't get many side effects on Herceptin. She was able to go back to work straight after her injections, and even did an all-night charity bike ride the day after one of her treatments.

Allergic reactions

Around 1 in 20 people have an allergic reaction during or up to 6 hours after their first Herceptin treatment. If this happens, you will feel unwell. Your lips may swell, you may feel breathless and develop a rash. You may also have a headache, dizziness or joint and muscle pains. If you think you're having an allergic reaction, tell your nurse immediately. If you're at home, you should call the emergency number you were given. You will be given medication to control the reaction and may be kept in hospital overnight.

Infection risk

Like chemotherapy, HER2 treatment lowers your immune system which means you are more likely to develop a serious infection. We tell you how to reduce your chances of developing an infection on page 147.

Heart damage

Herceptin, Perjeta and Tyverb can cause an abnormal heart rhythm or weaken a heart muscle called the left ventricle. This means your heart can't pump blood as well as it did before, which can make you tired, breathless or feel like your heart is fluttering. This complication occurs in a mild form in up to 20 per cent of patients and can cause serious long-term heart problems in around 2 per cent. Heart damage from Herceptin is more likely if you already had heart problems before treatment, such as a very high blood pressure, or are diabetic or overweight, though it can occur in previously fit people.

Before you start Herceptin, you will have a heart scan ('multiple-gated acquisition' or MUGA scan) to monitor how well your heart pumps. It is very similar to having an ultrasound scan and doesn't hurt. You lie on a couch while a doctor runs a probe over your chest to look at your heart muscle. It is repeated every 3–4 months throughout your treatment. If you do develop heart problems, these normally get better when Herceptin treatment stops, although a very small number of people are left with permanent heart damage.

> Trish's first heart scan showed a minor abnormality which was very alarming at the time. However, her oncologist reassured her that lots of healthy people have minor abnormalities found on heart scans which have no significance whatsoever. Her heart remained fine throughout her treatment, and this was confirmed with the repeated scans.

Sore mouth

Perjeta can give you a sore mouth which can be treated with a mild mouthwash, such as Difflam, and you should brush your teeth with a soft baby toothbrush.

Anaemia

Perjeta can also cause anaemia (not enough red blood cells) which can make you feel tired, weak and dizzy. The anaemia normally gets better once your treatment stops, but you might need an injection to stimulate your bone marrow (see page 133) or a blood transfusion to help.

OTHER TARGETED THERAPIES FOR SECONDARY BREAST CANCER

These are drugs given to patients with secondary breast cancer that target other specific proteins in (or on) cancer cells. They are used to complement chemotherapy drugs, which target all dividing cells. Some of them are only available as part of a research trial. New agents are being developed all the time, so this list may change in the future.

Palbociclib and Ribociclib (CDK4/6 inhibitors)

Palbociclib (Ibrance) and Ribociclib (Kisqali) block particular proteins called CDK4 and 6 enzymes. These affect cell growth and division. They are given to ER-positive patients, together with an Aromatase Inhibitor, and reduce the effects of oestrogen on cancer cells.

Everolimus

Everolimus (Afinitor) blocks a protein called mTOR which affects how cancer cells divide and grow. It is only given to patients with ER-positive secondary cancer resistant to hormonal therapy.

Bevacizumab

Bevacizumab (Avastin) interferes with how growing cancers develop their blood supply, and cuts off their supply of oxygen and food.

Targeted therapies are one of the most exciting new developments in the treatment of breast cancer, and we hope that in the future there will be even more drugs available to treat both primary and secondary breast cancer.

CHAPTER 12

RADIOTHERAPY

RADIOTHERAPY IS A cancer treatment that uses high-energy X-rays. The X-ray beams release pockets of energy as they pass through your body that damage and kill cancer cells. The X-rays also have an effect on healthy cells but most of these cells recover and repair themselves. Radiotherapy doesn't make you radioactive, and it's safe for you to be around pregnant women and children during your treatment.

If you have primary breast cancer, radiotherapy is given after you have finished surgery to reduce the risk of your cancer coming back and to improve your overall survival from breast cancer. If you have secondary cancer, radiotherapy is used to treat secondary deposits, for example in your brain or your bones, and for symptom control (see Chapter 23).

This chapter focuses on radiotherapy for primary breast cancer (for secondary cancer, see Chapter 23). There are four groups of people who will benefit:

After a lumpectomy

Radiotherapy reduces your risk of a local recurrence (cancer in the breast tissue, skin or chest wall muscles). Together with a lumpectomy, it gives the same risk of recurrence and survival as those women having a mastectomy. If you are under 50, or over 50 with a large or Grade 3 cancer, you may also be given an additional boost to the tumour bed (the area of your breast that surrounded the breast cancer) to further reduce the risk of recurrence.

After a mastectomy

You have a higher risk of getting a local recurrence if your cancer is large (over 4–5cm), Grade 3, has grown directly into the skin or the muscle underneath the breast, or if you have cancer in some of the lymph nodes in your armpit. Radiotherapy is given to your chest wall to reduce this risk.

After lymph node surgery

If you have cancer in four or more nodes, radiotherapy is given to the area above your collar bone (the 'supraclavicular fossa') to reduce the risk of local recurrence in the lymph nodes there. It may also be given if you have cancer in one to three axillary nodes and your cancer is large or a high-grade.

Instead of further lymph node surgery

If your sentinel lymph node biopsy was positive, your doctor may discuss radiotherapy to your armpit instead of further lymph node surgery. Trials have shown that surgery and radiotherapy are both equally effective at reducing the risk of recurrence. Your oncologist will help you decide which treatment to have.

QUESTIONS TO ASK YOUR ONCOLOGIST

- Why do I need radiotherapy?
- What are the side effects?
- Are there any alternative treatments?
- What might happen if I don't have it?
- How could it affect my surgery?
- What will my breast look like afterwards?

If you are over 70, with a small ER-positive, HER2-negative cancer and negative lymph nodes, your benefit from radiotherapy is small, and there are ongoing clinical trials investigating whether people like you can avoid radiotherapy.

When is radiotherapy given?

You have radiotherapy after you have recovered from your surgery, and ideally it should be given within a month or two after your surgery. It may have to be delayed if you have a wound infection, a large seroma that needs draining, you need further surgery or you can't lift your arms above your head. This is why it is important to do your shoulder exercises so your treatment isn't delayed. If you need to have chemotherapy, you will have this first, followed by radiotherapy once chemo has finished. If you are having Herceptin as well, your injections will continue while you have radiotherapy, and carry on until you have finished the course of treatment.

How is radiotherapy given?

Radiotherapy is measured in Grays (Gy). In the UK, most women get 40Gy given in 15 sessions over 3 weeks, from Monday to Friday. If you need a boost, this will involve an extra five to eight sessions. Most units run from early in the morning to late in the evening. You can ask for your sessions to be at a certain time to fit in around work and other commitments. You should be able to carry on working during treatment.

Most patients have External Beam Radiotherapy. The beams are delivered by a machine called a 'linear accelerator' (LINAC). Radiotherapy beams can also now be modulated (IMRT or Intensity-Modulated Radiotherapy) which means that stronger beams are sent to the target area, and the healthy surrounding tissues get a smaller dose. This can be done using the LINAC machine or another machine called a TomoTherapy machine.

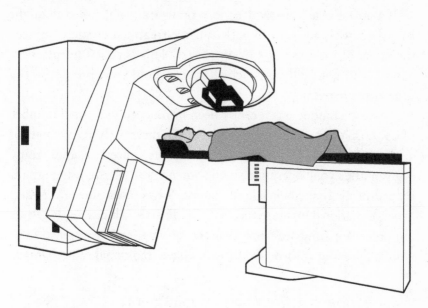

LINAC Machine

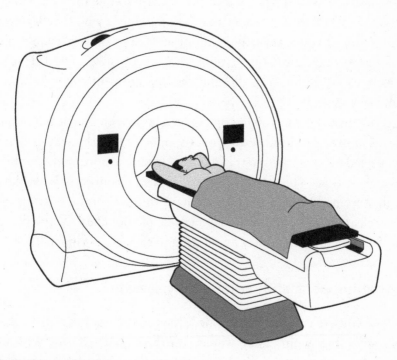

TomoTherapy Machine

If you have a left-sided cancer or heart problems you might be asked to hold your breath during treatment which reduces the effect of radiotherapy on the heart. This is called 'respiratory gating' and you will be coached how to hold your breath by the radiotherapy team.

A new technique has recently been introduced in a small number of UK hospitals called Intraoperative Radiotherapy (IORT) as part of a trial for women with small, node-negative cancers. Radiotherapy is given after your operation, while you are still asleep, using a ball-shaped probe that sits inside the breast. It has fewer side effects and avoids radiation damage to the skin, ribs, heart and lungs. Early results are promising, and we hope that the survival and recurrence rates will be the same as those women who have traditional radiotherapy.

What happens at your first appointment?

Your first appointment is a planning appointment for a CT scan to plan your radiotherapy and precisely map out the areas to be treated. You'll meet some of the radiotherapists who'll be looking after you. If you want female radiotherapists, you can ask at your planning scan, although it might not be possible. The CT scan takes 15–30 minutes to do, and the appointment can take up to an hour in total.

For the CT scan, you lie topless on a table with one or both your arms above your head resting on a support. Once the scan is done, you need to be marked so the radiotherapists can accurately position you each time. The marks are blue-black in colour, and look like a full-stop made with a pencil. You have three in total – one in your low cleavage area, and one on either side of your chest. You will feel a sharp scratch when they are done, and they are permanent.

What happens at a radiotherapy session?

Once you are correctly positioned, the radiotherapists will go into an adjoining room. They watch you through a window with an intercom so they can talk to you. Depending on which machine is being used, the machine will either move around you, or you may be moved inside the machine. It can be quite noisy, but it doesn't last for long – only five to ten minutes. Having radiotherapy is completely painless. You may find that the room is cold because of the air-conditioning. There will be blankets to put over your legs, but your arms may get cold.

> Liz used an old pair of thick woolly tights cut in two to keep her arms warm, with a pair of gloves for her hands as well.

It can be very emotional having radiotherapy. There is something quite unsettling about lying topless in a tunnel with your arms above your head in an empty room with nothing but your thoughts for company. However, each treatment only takes a couple of minutes, and the radiotherapists are wonderful at reassuring you and cheering you up afterwards. Liz even got hugs from hers.

Travelling to radiotherapy

Not every hospital has a radiotherapy department, and you might need to travel quite a distance, particularly if you live in a rural area. You may find the travelling exhausting, especially if you have to rely on public transport. If you drive, you may be entitled to reduced car parking charges, and this will be explained at your first appointment. If you're worried about how to get to the hospital, your doctor may be able to arrange hospital transport for you.

SIDE EFFECTS

Radiotherapy causes side effects that happen in the first few weeks and months of treatment (immediate), and some that happen several months or years later (late).

Immediate side effects
Skin reactions

These are very common after external beam radiotherapy, because the radiotherapy beams have to go through your skin to get to your breast. Your skin may become dry and sore, it might peel and flake, or turn red like a sunburn. Your skin can also change colour and darken like a deep suntan. Certain things make it worse, such as eczema, being overweight and smoking. You will be told to use non-perfumed moisturisers, soaps, shower gels and natural deodorants while you are having treatment, and for the first few weeks afterwards, until your skin settles down again. After radiotherapy, you are at a greater risk of getting burnt in the sun, so you should stay out of the sun during treatment and use a high factor sunscreen in the future. Wear loose clothing and you might want to stop wearing a bra for a while. Most skin reactions settle in a month or two.

Breast swelling

The breast can swell and feel tight and uncomfortable because of a build-up of fluid in the breast and skin. Regular breast massage can help: firmly rub your breast in a circular motion using a gentle moisturiser or non-perfumed massage oil for a couple of minutes every day.

Change in breast appearance

It is normal for your breast to change in size or shape after radiotherapy. Your breast may feel firm to the touch and shrink in size. There are surgical options to improve the look of your breast after radiotherapy, such as lipofilling (see page 99), but you'll have to wait at least 6–12 months until the final effects of radiotherapy have developed.

Shoulder stiffness

Your shoulder might feel sore, stiff and difficult to move, especially if you are having your armpit treated. You should keep doing your shoulder exercises for several months after radiotherapy has finished to combat this.

Sore throat and difficulty swallowing

If you've had your collarbone treated, you may get a sore throat and find it difficult to swallow for a couple of weeks. Simple pain-killers and throat sweets can help, as well as eating softer foods. This gets better after a week or two.

Chest pain

You may experience sharp aches or pains in your breast or chest wall which are normally mild and don't last very long. Sometimes these can continue for months or years, but should get better in time.

Hair loss

Radiotherapy causes your armpit hair (and chest hair, if you're a man) to fall out. It normally starts to grow back after a month or two, but sometimes it never grows back.

Late side effects

Arm swelling (lymphoedema)

If you have radiotherapy to the armpit, you can develop a swollen arm because the lymph nodes have been damaged. Lymphoedema is fully explained on page 96.

Change in breast shape after implant reconstruction

Radiotherapy can speed up the development of a capsule around your implant (see page 114). You may need surgery to correct this.

Skin changes

You may notice little red dots appearing on your skin due to tiny broken blood vessels. These are called 'telangiectasia'; they are harmless, but permanent.

Rib tenderness and fractures

Some people have tender ribs during treatment, and this can last for a long time. You may also be more likely to break a rib if you have an accident, so it's important to take extra care after treatment. If you do break a rib, the treatment is regular painkillers like paracetamol and ibuprofen to help with the pain and to let you take deep breaths, and the bone will repair itself over a couple of months.

Heart and lung problems

Sometimes, either due to your body shape or the position of the cancer within your breast, a small part of your heart and lungs may be damaged if they lie in the path of the X-ray beams, although newer techniques mean that your heart and lungs now receive very little radiation. There is a small chance that you might develop heart failure or inflammation of the lungs in the future. Your radiotherapy team will tell you if this applies to you, and also what signs to look out for.

Some people are scared of radiotherapy, but we hope we've been able to reassure you that it's not as bad as you think it is. It can be tiring, especially if you have to travel a long way for each session, so take it easy, and remember to look after your skin.

CHAPTER 13

HORMONE THERAPY AND OVARIAN SUPPRESSION

THE HORMONE OESTROGEN (or 'estrogen' in the USA, hence 'ER-positive') can stimulate the growth of some breast cancer cells. If you haven't gone through the menopause, you produce oestrogen in your ovaries. If you've had your menopause, or if you're a man, you still make some oestrogen in your body fat by converting other hormones using an enzyme called 'aromatase'.

As we said in Chapter 3, every breast cancer is tested to see whether it has oestrogen receptors. This is normally done from your core biopsy. An ER-positive (ER+ve) cancer has oestrogen receptors and is sensitive to oestrogen (about 85 per cent of all breast cancers worldwide). Liz's cancer was ER-positive, while Trish's was ER-negative. If you have an invasive ER-positive cancer, lowering the amount of oestrogen in your blood should stop your cancer growing and reduce the risk of it coming back in the future. If you have DCIS, you do not need this treatment because your cancer is non-invasive.

There are two ways to lower the amount of oestrogen in your body or the effect it has on your cells – hormone therapy and ovarian suppression – and these are discussed below.

HORMONE THERAPY

'Hormone therapy' means taking drugs to block the effects of oestrogen on breast cancer cells (like tamoxifen) or to stop you making oestrogen in your body fat (like an Aromatase Inhibitor).

Tamoxifen

Tamoxifen stops oestrogen attaching to breast cancer cells so they are no longer stimulated to grow. It is given to pre- and post-menopausal women with both primary and secondary breast cancer. Tamoxifen is a tablet that you take every day but it also comes as a liquid if you can't swallow tablets. It can harm your baby if you become pregnant, so you must use contraception while you are taking it.

Faslodex

Faslodex (fulvestrant) attaches to the oestrogen receptors and stops them working. It also reduces the number of receptors in the cancer cells. It is given to post-menopausal women with second-ary breast cancer whose cancer has progressed on other hormone therapies. It is given every two to four weeks as an injection in each buttock.

Aromatase Inhibitors

Aromatase Inhibitors (AIs) stop the enzyme aromatase making oestrogen in your body fat which lowers the amount of oestrogen in your body. They are given only to women who are post-meno-pausal with either primary or secondary breast cancer. If you are pre-menopausal, your ovaries are still producing oestrogen and therefore the AIs won't be anywhere near as effective for you.

There are three AIs, and they are all tablets that you take once a day:

1. Anastrazole (Arimidex)
2. Letrozole (Femara)
3. Exemestane (Aromasin)

When does hormone therapy start?
After surgery

You start taking hormone therapy when you have finished your chemotherapy and surgery. There are some research studies looking at the effect of giving hormone therapy before surgery, and your oncologist may talk to you about this if you are eligible to enter a trial. There is also some new evidence that some people could benefit from having hormonal therapy for several months before breast cancer surgery, but this is not currently done in the UK.

Instead of surgery

If your doctor doesn't think you are fit enough to have an operation and your cancer is ER-positive, they can treat you with hormonal therapy only. The aim is that it will shrink your cancer, or at least stop it growing. If it does start growing again, they may change you to a different tablet or reconsider surgery.

How long do you take hormonal therapy for?

We know that ER-positive breast cancer can come back after 10 or even 20 years. That is why you take hormone therapy for a long time. At the time of writing, if you have a low risk of recurrence, you will be advised to take hormone therapy for five years. If you have a higher risk of recurrence and are taking tamoxifen, recent trials have shown that taking it for another five years (ten years in total) further reduces the risk of your cancer coming back. The evidence is less clear if you are taking an AI. There may be some benefit in taking an AI for another two years (seven in total) or switching to tamoxifen for a further five years of treatment. Your doctor will see you in clinic after five years of treatment and advise you whether you need to stay on hormonal therapy, and how long for. New research findings are emerging all the time, so be prepared for the recommended time periods to change in the future.

Can you still use hormonal contraception and HRT with hormonal therapy?

Hormonal contraceptives (birth control pills and implants) and HRT (hormone replacement therapy) usually contain oestrogen. If your cancer is ER-positive, this oestrogen could stimulate it to grow and stop the hormone therapy from working. If you are currently taking the contraceptive pill or have an implant, you will need to switch to another form of contraception, such as a condom, cap or coil (see Chapter 17). If you are currently taking HRT, you must stop taking it before you can start hormone therapy.

QUESTIONS TO ASK YOUR DOCTOR

- Do I need hormone therapy?
- Will it improve my survival from breast cancer?
- How long will I need to take it for?
- Can I carry on taking HRT (hormone replacement therapy)?
- Can I still use the oral contraceptive pill or implant for contraception?
- What are the side effects?
- What happens if I can't cope with the side effects?
- Can I stop taking hormone therapy if I want to?

OVARIAN SUPPRESSION

If you are pre-menopausal, your oncologist may discuss stopping your ovaries working to further reduce the amount of oestrogen in your body and decrease the risk of recurrence. This also means that they can give you an AI, which might be more effective for your particular type of cancer. There are two ways to switch off your ovaries: drugs (like Zoladex) are used to stop your ovaries working, or you have an operation to remove your ovaries.

Drug treatment

Goserelin (Zoladex) is a drug that blocks the hormone that stimulates your ovaries to produce oestrogen. This means that you won't have periods any more, and will experience a sudden, early menopause. We explain this in more detail and tell you how to cope with menopausal symptoms in Chapter 16. Goserelin is given as a monthly injection into your tummy fat, just below the skin, either by a nurse in the hospital or a nurse in your GP surgery. Some patients may be able to eventually do it themselves. It is quite a large needle and can be uncomfortable or even painful to have, but the pain only lasts for a second or two. You may be offered an anaesthetic cream to put on the skin at home to help numb the area first. You'll be a little bruised and sore afterwards, and may notice a bit of bleeding at the injection site, but this is normal and nothing to worry about. The side effects of Goserelin are similar to the AIs (see page 172). When you stop Goserelin, your ovaries should start to work again.

Surgical treatment

Surgical removal of the ovaries is a permanent way to stop oestrogen production, and if you have this you will have a sudden, early menopause. If you have the BRCA gene (see page 3), you will be advised to have this operation once you are in your forties to stop you getting ovarian cancer. It is a keyhole operation with a general anaesthetic where the surgeon uses a camera connected to a screen to look inside your tummy, and uses small instruments to remove your ovaries. You will be left with a few small scars low on your tummy, and one in your belly button where the camera goes in.

QUESTIONS TO ASK YOUR DOCTOR

- Do I need ovarian suppression?
- Will it improve my survival from breast cancer?
- What is the difference between an injection and surgery?
- What are the side effects?
- Is it reversible?

SIDE EFFECTS

All of the therapies above have a large number of potential side effects, mainly menopausal, which most of you will experience to a certain degree. They tend to get better over time, generally within a year of starting the therapy.

With hormonal therapy, some patients say that one brand of tablet gives them fewer side effects compared to another. If you are finding it hard to cope, you could ask your pharmacist to order you a different brand to try. We know that some patients don't take their tablets regularly because of the side effects, but few of them admit this to their doctor. We do understand that the side effects can be hard to deal with, and Liz still struggles with some of them. However, if you don't take the tablets, you are increasing the chance that your cancer might come back in the future.

If you are struggling with the side effects, please talk to your doctor before discontinuing. They can use the PREDICT tool (see page 31) to calculate your individual benefit from hormone therapy. If it is very small, maybe 1–2 per cent, this means that if 100 women have hormone therapy, only one or two of them will live longer because of it, and this might make it easier for you to decide to stop taking your tablets. However, if your estimated benefit is much greater, say 5–10 per cent, you might decide it is worth coping with the side effects to reduce the risk of your cancer coming back.

Menopausal symptoms

You may not have any menopausal symptoms, especially if your own menopause was some time ago. However, it can be completely different if you are pre-menopausal and suddenly thrown into an instant early menopause, like Liz was. One day Liz was 'normal', and the next she was stripping off in supermarkets and waking up in the middle of the night thinking she had wet herself, thanks to hot flushes and night sweats. It was a huge shock to the system, and it took her several months to get used to it. We talk about menopausal symptoms and, more importantly, how to cope with them in Chapter 16.

Bone thinning

If you have had ovarian suppression or are taking an AI, you may be at risk of osteoporosis (bone thinning). This is discussed in more detail on page 179.

Blood clots

A rare but potentially fatal side effect of hormone therapy is developing a blood clot in a vein in your leg (DVT or Deep Vein Thrombosis). This starts as a painful, swollen calf and you should see your doctor urgently if you develop this. If it's not treated, the clot can spread to your lungs (PE or Pulmonary Embolism). This causes chest pain and shortness of breath and is very serious. If you need to have an operation in the future, you must tell your surgeon that you are taking hormone therapy, because an operation can cause a DVT. They will probably ask you to stop taking it for two to four weeks before your operation to reduce the risk of you getting a blood clot after the surgery.

High blood pressure and cholesterol

Hormone therapy can raise your blood pressure and the cholesterol level in your blood. If you already have a high blood pressure or a high cholesterol level, you should ask your GP whether you need extra monitoring or treatment.

Fluid build-up and leg cramps

Low oestrogen levels can make you hold on to water in your tissues. About 1 in 10 women develop swollen ankles, legs and fingers. You may also get cramps in your legs. Regular exercise and support socks/tights can help, but you may have to tolerate swollen legs for the duration of your treatment.

Carpal tunnel syndrome

This is a condition characterised by tingling, weakness and (occasionally) pain in your hand. It is caused by fluid build-up in the tissues at your wrist which causes a nerve to become squashed. It is normally treated with a wrist support. If this doesn't work you may need a steroid injection or a small operation to fix it.

Hair thinning and hair loss

Your hair may start to thin. Be gentle with it, brush and comb it gently, and try to avoid using hair straighteners and curling tongs. It should go back to normal once you stop taking hormone therapy.

Additional side effects of tamoxifen

The following side effects can also occur with tamoxifen:

- *Endometrial cancer:* Tamoxifen can thicken the lining of your womb (endometrium), which can give you unexpected vaginal bleeding or pain, and you may need to have treatment for it. Very rarely, the thickening can develop into a cancer of your womb. If you do get unusual bleeding, you should see your GP to get it checked out.

- *Stomach problems:* You may get indigestion or feel slightly sick when you first start taking tamoxifen. This normally gets better in time.
- *Eye problems:* Rarely, tamoxifen can cause blurring of your vision (a cataract), changes in your eyesight or changes in the back of your eye. You should tell your optician that you are taking tamoxifen – they may recommend an eye test every year.

Additional side effects of AIs

The following side effects can also occur with AIs:

- *Joint and muscle pain:* This is one of the most common side effects. Most people have pain in the joints of their fingers, hands and feet, and this may be worse if you already have arthritis. The pain can normally be controlled with paracetamol, but you may need to switch to tamoxifen if it doesn't get any better.
- *Headaches, nausea, vomiting and loss of appetite:* You may experience some or all of these, and they usually get better with time. Paracetamol can help with the headaches. If you can't cope with feeling sick, your GP may be able to give you a tablet to help. Try taking your tablets with or after food and eat small, frequent meals and snacks.
- *Dizziness.* This is a rare side effect. If you feel dizzy, you shouldn't drive. It normally gets better in time, but if it doesn't, you should see your GP.

BONE HEALTH

Oestrogen strengthens your bones. After the menopause, when your ovaries stop producing oestrogen, your bones start to weaken and thin. This is called 'osteoporosis'. When you have an AI or ovarian suppression, this can increase the rate at which your bones thin, because you have less oestrogen. If your bones remain weak, you are more likely to break your bones (e.g. your wrist, hip or spine) if you have a fall. Tamoxifen doesn't have the same effect because it doesn't lower your levels of oestrogen; it just stops it attaching to breast cancer cells.

How do you know how strong your bones are?

Before you have either an AI or ovarian suppression, you will have a bone density (DEXA) scan to measure your bone strength. This is a very quick scan which involves lying on a table while an X-ray is taken of your back and one of your hips. The DEXA scan is normally repeated every couple of years while you are on treatment.

Your DEXA scan produces a T-score and a Z-score. The T-score compares your bone strength with that of a healthy young adult. The Z-score compares your bone strength with an average person of your age. If your scores are low, it means that your bones are weaker than an average person, and you need treatment to help stop them thinning further.

How is osteoporosis treated?
Diet

Your bones rely on calcium to stay strong, and your body needs vitamin D to be able to use the calcium in your diet. You make vitamin D when you are out in the sun, but you might not make enough if you spend a lot of time indoors or live in a country where there isn't a lot of sunshine. Most people get enough calcium in their diet from dairy foods, green vegetables, soya products and tinned fish. Your doctor may recommend that you take a daily calcium and vitamin D supplement to help keep your bones strong. You should cut down on caffeine and alcohol and try to stop smoking, as all of these can weaken your bones.

Exercise

Regular weight-bearing exercise is really important to help keep your bones strong. It is why most active people don't get osteoporosis when they are older. Weight-bearing exercise is when you support your own body weight, for example walking, climbing the stairs, running, aerobics and tennis, but not swimming (see Chapter 18 for more on this).

Bisphosphonates

A bisphosphonate (such as Alendronate or Fosamax) is a drug that strengthens your bones. If you are taking an AI, you may be advised to take a bisphosphonate as well to stop your bones thinning. There is also some new evidence to show that bisphosphonates can reduce the risk of getting recurrent breast cancer in your bones, so your doctor may advise taking it even if you are not on an AI.

You must see your dentist before you start taking bisphosphonates, especially if you need to have teeth extracted or major dental work done. Bisphosphonates can weaken your jaw bone, and there is a very, very small chance that your jaw bone might not heal after dental surgery and could even start to die. This is very difficult to treat, but it is rare.

Bisphosphonates are normally given as a tablet which you take either every day or once a week. Your stomach has to be empty before you take it, so you take it either first thing in the morning before you have had anything to eat or drink, or at least six hours after you last ate or drank. Because the drugs can damage the lining of your gullet, you then have to stay sitting upright or standing for at least half an hour after you have taken them, and wait at least half an hour before having anything else to eat or drink, or taking any other tablets. If you are struggling to take the tablets, your doctor may be able to prescribe you a bisphosphonate injection instead, which is given either monthly, three- or six-monthly.

As you can see, hormone therapy and ovarian suppression have a lot of side effects that many people have trouble dealing with. However, there is a lot of evidence that proves they greatly reduce the risk of your cancer coming back. You should now understand why it is so important to have this treatment, and we hope we have reassured you that the side effects do get better in time. If you are struggling to cope, please talk things through with your doctor.

CHAPTER 14

WHERE TO GET SUPPORT

GOING THROUGH CANCER treatment can be bewildering and stressful. It can be hard to know where to turn to get the information and support that you need, and some of the information you find may do more harm than good. We want to show you where you can get the help you need. Many of the resources described in this chapter are Internet-based. If you've never used the Internet, you may need to ask a friend or family member to show you how. Alternatively, you could use a library or ask a friend to print things out for you.

DROP-IN CANCER CENTRES

Cancer centres, or drop-in centres, are usually run by a voluntary sector organisation and are based in or near large hospitals. They have been designed to meet the different needs of patients and families going through cancer treatment. They are open to anyone affected by cancer and their family, at any time during treatment or even years later. No appointment is needed.

In the UK, the leading chain of hospital-based drop-in centres are Maggie's Centres – their website tells you which hospitals have them: www.maggiescentres.org. Macmillan have a drop-in centre in most hospitals, although these are normally small information hubs. There are also the UK-wide Jewish Chai Cancer Care centres and local Christian cancer centres. Breast Cancer Haven has centres across the UK offering specific support for people affected by breast cancer. Finally, there are Penny's centres and the Big C centres. (See the resources list on page 276 for more details.) There may be others local to you.

Why might you go to a drop-in centre?

Drop-in centres are a welcoming friendly place in what can otherwise feel like a hostile hospital environment. They have free tea, coffee and biscuits, and there is always someone to talk to, whether you are a patient or a relative. They understand what it's like to live with cancer and know how hard it can feel. People will be nice to you there – and sometimes that can mean a lot in itself. They can be a better place than a hospital café for your relative or friend to wait while you are having tests or treatments.

In addition, most drop-in centres offer complementary therapies, one-to-one and group support, counselling, gentle exercise and mindfulness classes, and beauty classes for patients, and most of these are free. If there is a drop-in centre near you, we strongly encourage you to pop in for a cup of tea before you go home, and take advantage of everything they offer. If you don't have one near you, like us, your cancer nurse should be able to tell you if similar courses, classes and therapies are run locally, and give you information so you can attend them.

Here are some of the courses offered in drop-in centres:

'Look Good Feel Better'

This is a two- to three-hour class for cancer patients designed to improve your well-being and help you feel more confident about your appearance. Trained beauty consultants sit with a small number of you and go through skincare and make-up products, and show you how to apply them. If you have lost your eyebrows and eyelashes due to chemo, they will show you how to draw them on, which can be challenging when there is no hair to guide you. You are sent home with a large bag of skincare products, perfume and make-up, which is an added bonus.

Group support

In group support sessions, you meet regularly (typically once a week) with other patients in a similar situation to you. Your partner may be invited to join too. You talk about whatever you like – it doesn't have to be cancer-related – and a facilitator sits in the session to help lead and support the group. Research shows that group support can reduce psychological distress and improve quality of life in people with cancer, especially if you don't have a close supportive relationship in your personal life.

Individual peer support

Here you are paired with someone who has been through the same diagnosis or a similar set of treatments to you. Whereas the doctors and nurses can tell you what will happen to you, your peer supporter (sometimes referred to as your 'cancer buddy') will tell you what it's really like to have each treatment. They will give you tips for weathering the storm, and this can be invaluable.

Professional counselling

This is one-on-one support with a psychologist or trained counsellor. Most cancer units have access to a psychologist who is used to treating cancer patients and their unique set of needs and concerns. Some people find this kind of professional support extremely helpful in dealing with cancer-related stress.

Mindfulness and meditation

Mindfulness and meditation encourage you to focus on the present moment and your five senses (sight, sound, touch, taste and smell) while you concentrate on your breathing. This means you naturally 'zone out' from distractions, fears, negative thoughts and things *not* immediately present. If negative thoughts do enter your mind, you learn to acknowledge them and let them go, instead of dwelling on them. It only takes a few minutes every day, and can help you feel calm and in control again. There is now strong research evidence that mindfulness can reduce symptoms of stress in women with breast cancer.

Most drop-in centres run mindfulness and meditation classes. Alternatively, you could do it yourself at home. Liz used the app 'Headspace', which guides you through a short daily meditation. We also liked the book *Mindfulness: A Kindly Approach to Being with Cancer* by Dr Trish Bartley (Wiley-Blackwell, 2016).

COMPLEMENTARY THERAPIES

These are therapies intended to *complement,* not replace, your conventional medical treatment for breast cancer. They can make your cancer experience easier by reducing your stress and improving your well-being. It's also lovely to let someone pamper you occasionally.

There is no good scientific evidence that complementary therapies improve your chance of surviving cancer. If you do choose to use them *instead of* normal breast cancer treatments, this could seriously reduce your chances of long-term survival and lead to an early death.

Massage

Massage can make you feel better generally and is said to improve the lymphatic circulation. If you were used to having firm massage treatments before you got breast cancer, we suggest you have a light, relaxing massage the first time. There are many different kinds of massage:

- *Swedish massage*: a medium-intensity full-body massage.
- *Chinese massage*: includes deep-tissue massage focusing on channels or 'energy points' similar to acupuncture points.

- *Shiatsu*: a Japanese massage technique that can be high-intensity.
- *Deep tissue massage*: works on removing 'knots' and relieving long-standing tension.
- *Aromatherapy massage*: a massage therapy with nice-smelling oils (see page 188).
- *Reflexology*: specialised foot massage using 'energy points'.

Most cancer centres offer massage treatments without question, but the experience may be different to a massage salon on the high street. For insurance purposes, most salon therapists need you to get a letter from your doctor saying that it is safe for you to have a massage. This can be very annoying (Liz was turned away in tears during chemotherapy because she didn't realise she needed a letter). You should probably wait for several weeks after your surgery or radiotherapy before you have a massage, and make sure your therapist knows which treatment you have had so they can tailor your massage accordingly.

Acupuncture

Acupuncture is an ancient Chinese therapy in which a practitioner inserts very fine needles into the skin at key points on the body. The needles stimulate nerves beneath the skin, causing the body to produce natural chemicals called endorphins that give you a feeling of well-being and work as a natural painkiller.

Some research studies have shown that acupuncture can help reduce chemotherapy-related side effects (such as nausea, aches and pains, and insomnia) and help with severe hot flushes, but these studies aren't particularly high-quality. Acupuncture won't do you any harm, as long as it is carried out by a skilled practitioner who uses sterile, clean needles and knows to avoid the arm on the side of any lymph node surgery.

Trish once tried acupuncture for migraine; the acupuncturist was charming and the experience was not unpleasant, but it didn't cure the migraine.

Aromatherapy

Aromatherapy uses plant-derived fragrant oils to stimulate your sense of smell, which aromatherapists believe helps healing, although there is very little scientific evidence to prove this. It is often combined with massage, and can be a great way to relax if you like the scents used.

Energy therapies

These include Reiki, therapeutic touch and spiritual healing. They are meant to restore your well-being by unblocking energy channels and letting healing energy flow through you. Neither of us has tried these, and we are both a little sceptical. However, if you want to try them to help you heal, there is no harm in having them during your cancer treatment.

CANCER CHARITIES

There are three main UK cancer charities that can help anyone with breast cancer. The most well-known resource for patients with any type of cancer (and their relatives) is Macmillan Cancer Support, a large UK-based charity whose motto is 'no one facing cancer should walk alone'. Their extensive range of resources (both online materials and printed booklets), the much-valued Macmillan helpline (human support on the end of the phone) and face-to-face support where needed, are free. Macmillan know that cancer affects every aspect of your life – from the way you look to the impact on your family finances – and, as they say, they're there to help. You will find their free leaflets in the waiting room of your cancer centre, which you can also download to send to family and friends.

The charity Breast Cancer Care is a similar resource aimed at patients with primary or secondary breast cancer, and their families. They also have many information leaflets about breast cancer treatments and coping with cancer that you may be given by your breast care nurse. You can also download these online. They offer a fantastic free service called 'Someone Like Me' where you can email or talk to a trained volunteer who has also had breast cancer and knows exactly what you are going through.

The charity Breast Cancer Now is the UK's leading breast cancer research charity, and they also offer information about breast cancer treatment and help you understand what is happening to you. See pages 277–80 for contact details for these charities.

ONLINE SUPPORT GROUPS

In the UK, both Macmillan and Breast Cancer Care have online forums where you can talk to other cancer patients about topics that matter to you. You don't have to use your own name, and the forums are moderated. This means that someone checks the postings and gives the discussion a steer when needed, for example, suggesting that the content or tone of a thread is inappropriate. Trish used a forum on the American charity website BreastCancer.org. All the forums have groups for patients starting treatment in a specific month, whether that is surgery or radiotherapy, so you can talk to people having treatment at the same time as you and support each other through it. Trish felt a huge sense of relief as her group ticked off the early milestones (that first chemo visit was horrible, but it didn't kill us) and the forum brought pragmatism and a sense of humour to the daily grind of cancer treatment.

There are many other websites with online forums (see for example Inspire: www.inspire.com). Feel free to explore and find one that works for you. However, some forums may not be moderated, which means that people can post misinformation or potentially hurtful comments without being checked. Because of this, we'd recommend sticking to the forums listed above. If you do use a different forum, do a bit of exploring on the site first to make sure that it feels right for you.

SOCIAL MEDIA

'Social media' means using the Internet or applications such as Twitter, Facebook, Snapchat and WhatsApp to stay in touch and reach out to people. If you don't use any of these sites, please don't worry. If you do, you may want to use them as a means of gaining information and support.

Twitter

We are both active twitter users. Liz (@Liz_ORiordan) 'came out' on Twitter the day after she was diagnosed and found a whole new world of friendly breast cancer patients who shared their tips and tricks to cope with treatment, in effect creating her own public forum. Trish (@trishgreenhalgh) didn't tell people. Instead, she used Twitter to get information and support about breast cancer by following people and organisations who tweeted about the condition. To get you started, we recommend following Macmillan (@macmillancancer), Breast Cancer Care (@bccare), Breast Cancer Now (@breastcancernow), Breast Cancer Chat Worldwide (@bccww) and After Breast Cancer Diagnosis (@abcdi-agnosis). For men, we suggest the Male Breast Cancer Coalition (@MBCC_MHBT).

To get a head start at finding people who tweet a lot about breast cancer, you could join a 'tweetchat'. This is an hour-long discussion every week led by patients that focuses on a different topic each time. The hashtags to follow are #bccww in the UK (9pm, Tuesdays) and #bcsm in America (9pm Eastern time, Mondays). You can also get information about the latest developments in breast cancer treatment, since many doctors and patients now live-tweet from scientific conferences and share the key points.

Facebook

If you use Facebook, you could join Breast Cancer Care's online Facebook community (breastcancercare). There is a private community called 'YBCN' for young women with breast cancer, and one called 'Flat Friends' for women who have had a double mastectomy. Spend some time searching for groups that you like the look of.

> We can't stress enough how important our online support was in helping us get through breast cancer and chemotherapy. Being able to swear, laugh and cry about everything that is happening to you, with someone who understands exactly what you are going through, can be lifesaving.

One thing that we have learned is that having cancer can be lonely. You may not meet another breast cancer patient during your treatment, and it can be very hard to know whether the physical symptoms and emotions you are feeling are normal. Getting support from people who understand what you're going through, whether it's from a cancer centre, a therapist or other patients, can make a huge difference to your well-being.

CHAPTER 15

COPING WITH CHANGES
TO YOUR BODY

BREAST CANCER TREATMENT will inevitably change how your body looks. Some of the changes are obvious, such as hair loss, but others are only seen by you, such as your surgical scars. These body changes can be unnerving. Many women also gain weight because of chemotherapy and the menopause, and all of these changes can be a daily reminder that you have had breast cancer. We want to help you cope with the changes that your body goes through, and this chapter will cover everything from why you are more likely to gain weight than lose it, to body image and how to get used to being a different shape and size.

WEIGHT

Weight gain during and after breast cancer treatment is common, due to the side effects (physical and mental) of treatment. Hormone therapy (see Chapter 13) can bring on the menopause (Chapter 16), and weight gain is a well-known side effect. Chemotherapy (Chapter 10) can make you feel lethargic, and because you are spending more time in hospital than women who just had surgery and radiotherapy, you may end up eating a lot of junk food in hospital cafés. Chemotherapy can also make you feel sick, and many women constantly snack to relieve this. Visitors bring you chocolate as a treat, and, finally, having cancer is miserable so it's tempting to comfort eat.

Here's the dilemma. On the one hand, cancer treatment is really tough, so you shouldn't beat yourself up if you put on a bit of weight. On the other hand, research has shown that the more overweight you are, the more likely you are to get a recurrence of your breast cancer. If you gain a lot of weight during cancer treatment it can be very hard to lose it afterwards. It also increases your risk of developing heart disease, high blood pressure and type 2 diabetes. Though we realise that this is easier said than done, you can keep your weight under control by being sensible about what and how much you eat, and being as active as you can. We go through this in more detail in Chapter 18.

Not everyone gains weight during treatment. There is no better way of controlling your weight than watching what you eat and increasing the amount of activity you do each day. Despite this, you may find it impossible to shift the extra pounds, and it can be hard to learn to accept your new body, especially with all the other changes that have happened. Be kind to yourself, and we hope you will learn to love your body at its new shape and weight.

> The hospital unit where Trish had her chemo provided excellent home-made cakes, but she felt she had to 'earn' the treat by doing a long power walk before her treatment!
>
> Liz suffered with very bad sickness during chemo, and would lose 2–3kg in the first few days which she put back on again before the next treatment.

FATIGUE AND DECONDITIONING

One of the most common side effects of cancer and its treatment is fatigue. This is different from simply feeling tired. Fatigue can influence your mood, your relationship and your ability to work (both inside and outside the home), not to mention restricting your ability to go out and socialise.

Everyone gets tired from time to time – after strenuous activity, at the end of a long day or after a visit to certain relatives. Fatigue happens when (for example):

- You have tiredness that is not related to physical exertion.
- Your tiredness rarely goes away or keeps returning, however much rest or sleep you have.
- You feel weak, as if (as Trish's mum used to say) you 'couldn't pull the skin off a rice pudding'.
- You are sleeping more than usual and/or have difficulty sleeping.
- Your tiredness is associated with feeling confused, lacking concentration or inability to focus your thoughts.
- You feel irritable, sad or depressed as well as tired.

If you have any of the above symptoms, tell your doctor. They may want to do some simple tests to make sure nothing else is wrong. A blood test can find a treatable cause, such as anaemia, an underactive thyroid or even heart failure (though this is not common).

The most likely cause, however, is that the fatigue is a side effect of your cancer treatment, perhaps combined with you becoming deconditioned (out of shape, with loss of muscle strength, flexibility and balance) as a result of being ill. Your GP may be able to change your current medication (for example, some antihistamines have a strong sedative effect while others don't), or you may need treatment for depression (see Chapter 4 for advice on this).

It can help to keep a diary of when the fatigue occurs and what it feels like. Are there any 'triggers'? Are you worse on days when you do less exercise or more exercise? Is your fatigue linked to alcohol? Is the fatigue associated with pain? (If so, ask for a review of your painkillers.) If your fatigue is simply because you have had cancer, it can be hard to treat. Karen Mullin and her colleagues recently reviewed all the research literature on this condition for *Lancet Oncology* (2017; 3: 961). They found that both exercise therapy and psychological therapy were effective in reducing fatigue and that, compared to these, medication was less effective.

If just the thought of exercise is exhausting, use 'baby steps': it doesn't matter how little you do, just do *something* and build from that. Walk to the nearest lamp post and back. Tomorrow, try two and build the distance gradually. You could also try some strengthening exercises to tighten and tone your muscles. Use two tins of food (such as baked beans) as hand weights; curl them up to your chin and then slowly down to touch your thighs and repeat 10 times. If your home has stairs, step up onto the first step and down again. Repeat 10 times. If 10 is too easy, try 20. If 10 is too hard, try 5. We talk more about exercise in Chapter 18.

Psychological therapy includes mindfulness and cognitive behavioural therapy, which we cover in Chapter 14. It's important to be open to the possibility that a physical condition like fatigue may respond to mental 'exercises'. Yoga (described on page 236) can include both physical exercise and mindfulness techniques.

At the same time as trying to improve your stamina, develop tactics to live within your means. Ask for help and prioritise tasks (and people). Plan your day so you have a balance of physical activity, something socially strenuous and rests in between. If a heavy day is coming up, plan a rest day the day before and after. Stop activities before you become too tired – you simply won't be able to 'push through it'.

As we explain in Chapter 18, we recommend that you eat sensibly, with a focus on eating the right amount of healthy, fresh food.

Finally, don't feel bad if you can't finish things you would have achieved easily before cancer or if you become 'dependent' on friends and neighbours. And play the cancer card when necessary.

BODY IMAGE

Breast cancer treatment can make you look and feel very different. As well as possible weight gain, you will have scars from your biopsies and surgeries and your breasts may be a different shape, be numb to the touch or you may no longer have them. Radiotherapy may have left you with skin damage, and if you lost your hair during chemotherapy, you may have to cope with having hair that grows back with a different texture or colour.

No wonder many women feel ugly, lop-sided, unfeminine, unfit, incomplete – even freakish – after treatment. On top of this, few women are 100 per cent happy with their bodies before they get cancer. You may not want to look in a mirror, get undressed in front of your partner or show your scars in a communal changing room. This reaction is normal and understandable, but please be assured that those feelings do improve in time. Research has shown that at two years after diagnosis, only 15–30 per cent of women still have concerns. Long-term problems with body image are more common in younger women, those who are overweight and those who have had more radical surgery or a delayed reconstruction.

The charity Breast Cancer Care has an excellent guide 'Your body, intimacy and sex' which says:

> Research has shown that the sooner you confront the physical changes to your body, the easier you may find it to gain confidence in the way you look ... If you have a partner, letting them see the surgical scars and changes to your body sooner may also make being intimate easier in the long term. The first few times you look at yourself might make you feel unhappy and shocked, and you may want to avoid looking at yourself again. However, the initial intense feelings you may have will lessen over time as you get more used to how you look now.

The tips below, which are mentioned in the guide, are adapted from 'Intimacy and sexuality for cancer patients and their partners' (available at sexualadviceassociation.co.uk). You should work through this sequence slowly. There's no hurry – and nothing will be gained from trying to force the pace if you're finding it difficult.

- *Start fully clothed.* Put on an outfit you like, and look at yourself in a full-length mirror. Pick out three things you really like about yourself.

- *Now try it in underwear.* Find a comfortable set of underwear (or a swimsuit) and practice looking at yourself with most of your flesh showing. Is it really that bad? This is more than most people are even going to see of you.
- *The naked view.* When you feel ready, move on to looking at your naked body in a full-length mirror. Describe what you see. Think about what you like about your body – and about what makes you feel awkward or uncomfortable.
- *Focus on the changes.* When you can look at your whole body naked, you are ready to start exploring what's happened to your body. Look at your scars and breast reconstruction. Touch them so you get used to how they feel.
- *Keep doing all of the above.* The more often you look at and feel your body, the less different it will seem.

Here are some additional tips from us on how to improve your body image:

- *Work on your weight.* You won't be able to bring back a breast or a nipple that's been removed, but you can take control of your body size. We know it's not easy – but it's not impossible.
- *Work on your fitness.* Knowing your body is strong and healthy can help you appreciate what it can do for you, and by toning up muscle, you will look better too. Keeping fit will also reduce the risk of recurrence (see Chapter 18).
- *Try mindfulness exercises.* You can train your mind to stop focusing on negative thoughts (see Chapter 14).
- *Treat yourself.* Have a manicure, a pedicure or a massage. Buy a new lipstick. Get a really good haircut. These little things can really help you feel good.
- *Think about body art.* In addition to a conventional nipple tattoo (designed to make your nipple look like a normal nipple), you may want to have an artistic tattoo to cover your scars. This can be really empowering. Remember that a tattoo is permanent and it can become infected, so think carefully

before choosing this option. For ideas, see the US website
P.ink or the tattoo section of Breast Cancer Care.

- *Ask to be referred for counselling or psychotherapy.* If your
body image problems are severe, you may need professional
help to move forward. Most therapists will use a variant of
cognitive behavioural therapy with some success.
- *Plan and work on a new 'look'.* Perhaps get your hair restyled
or recoloured (wait at least six months after the end of chemo
to do this). Go clothes shopping with a friend and reinvent
yourself. Try stuff on that you wouldn't have tried before.
The 'Look Good Feel Better' programme (see Chapter 14)
can help you experiment with make-up. Be bold. Have fun.
You're different now – own it.

On a final note, here's a quote from Breast Cancer Care's policy
report 'My body, myself', written by a young woman who had had
a mastectomy:

Dear Body

I wasn't always happy with you. I wanted longer legs, a flatter
tummy, firmer arms. But recently we've been through a lot, you
and I. We've faced cancer, together. We lost our right breast. Our
hair fell out. But we got through it. And now I've learned to love
and accept you for what you are. Not perfect, but beautifully
imperfect. You are my body. And I'm proud of you.

CHAPTER 16

TREATMENT-INDUCED MENOPAUSE AND INFERTILITY

MENOPAUSAL SYMPTOMS OCCUR when the level of oestrogen in your body drops. Hormonal therapy, ovarian suppression and chemotherapy all reduce the amount of oestrogen in your body, and they can also affect your future fertility.

MENOPAUSE

Being thrown into a sudden menopause because of chemotherapy or hormonal manipulation is much harder to cope with than a natural menopause because it happens overnight, instead of a gradual build-up over several years. Trish had already gone through the menopause when she started treatment, but Liz hadn't, and she found it very hard to deal with, on top of chemotherapy and a mastectomy. Above all, she hated feeling old before her time. We're going to walk you through what the menopause is, and how to cope if it happens to you.

What is the menopause?

The menopause is when you stop having periods and can no longer have a baby, and normally starts in your early fifties. It happens because your ovaries slowly stop producing the hormones oestrogen and progesterone, and takes several years. Your body undergoes several changes because of the low oestrogen levels which can cause a wide variety of symptoms (explained on pages 202–5).

How does breast cancer treatment affect the menopause?

Chemotherapy, ovarian suppression and hormone therapy can cause an immediate early menopause if you are young or may worsen your symptoms if you are already menopausal. The symptoms are more intense if your menopause is immediate, unlike a natural menopause when your body has several years to adjust. It can be very hard to cope at first, especially if you are young and faced with a daily reminder that you've had breast cancer. The symptoms normally get better within a year or two. Going through the menopause can also affect your partner and your relationship. It's important to talk to them and explain why you are getting menopausal symptoms so they know what it happening to you and why.

Trish was 56 and post-menopausal when she got breast cancer. She'd been taking hormone replacement therapy (HRT) to control her symptoms. When her breast cancer was diagnosed, she was advised to stop HRT. This brought back troublesome symptoms, especially hot flushes, which settled down after a few weeks. Her GP prescribed her some oestrogen pessaries to help with vaginal dryness.

Liz was 40 when she was diagnosed and was thrown into an instant menopause with chemotherapy, which continued on tamoxifen. Like most young women, she found it very hard to cope and thought things would never settle down. It took a good couple of years for her symptoms to improve, but they are slowly getting better now.

How do you know if you're menopausal?

Your doctor can check this with a blood test to monitor the levels of two hormones:

1. *Follicle-stimulating hormone (FSH)* is made by the brain. It stimulates your ovaries to produce eggs. As the menopause approaches, the ovaries stop responding and the brain makes more FSH. Therefore, *high* levels of FSH (about 100 times higher than a pre-menopausal woman) indicate you are menopausal.
2. *Estradiol (or oestrodiol)* is the main form of oestrogen found in your blood. If you are pre-menopausal, you will have high levels, but after the menopause these levels will fall to less than one-tenth of their previous levels.

HORMONE REPLACEMENT THERAPY (HRT)

HRT is a treatment often given to women to help them cope with the menopause by replacing oestrogen and/ or progesterone. If your cancer is sensitive to oestrogen, you will be strongly advised not to take HRT because it increases your oestrogen levels, which will increase your risk of recurrence and your risk of developing breast cancer in your other breast. If your symptoms are so severe that they are affecting your quality of life, it may be worth the risk of taking HRT while accepting that it might make your cancer come back. Only you can decide whether you want to take that chance.

If your cancer isn't sensitive to oestrogen, your oncologist may say it's okay to take a low dose of HRT for a short time to control the worst of the symptoms. There is a risk, however, that HRT will increase your chance of developing a second breast cancer that is sensitive to oestrogen.

Menopausal symptoms
Hot flushes and night sweats

These are the most common and (often) the most troublesome symptoms. They happen when the sluggish ovary releases a little burst of oestrogen. Most women get a couple of flushes every day but you can get them two to three times every hour, day and night. They range from a mild sensation of warmth in your face to a full body flush that leaves you dripping in sweat, then shivering as the sweat dries. They can be embarrassing and distressing, especially if they happen in public. They normally last for a few seconds, and can be triggered by spicy food, alcohol and caffeine.

Night sweats can mean you wake up on wet sheets. They can affect your sex life (as bodily contact can bring them on), and you may find yourself pushing your partner away. They can disturb your sleep, leaving you feeling tired and irritable, and you may forget things or find it harder to concentrate as a result. Your partner may also get less sleep as you wake them up when you fling your bedcovers on the floor.

> Menopausal symptoms can sometimes be unexpected. When Liz first had a night sweat, she thought she had wet herself because she felt liquid trickling down her inner thigh.

Here are our tips to help you cope:

- *Avoid triggers.* Keep a diary to see if you can identify anything that brings them on.
- *Clothing.* Wear layers so you can easily strip off when you get a hot flush. At night, try wearing sports clothes that wick away sweat. Natural fibres (cotton and silk) might keep you cooler than man-made fibres (such as nylon and polyester). Mattress

and pillow protectors will stop sheets getting stained. If you have a partner, try using two single duvets so they don't get disturbed when you throw off the cover. You can then use a lighter weight duvet if you want.

- *Accessories.* Carry a small hand or battery-operated fan in your handbag and a water spray for your face. You can also buy gel pillows or 'chillows' that stay icy cold which are wonderful when you're having a night sweat.
- *Complementary therapies.* Acupuncture, hypnotherapy, massage and reflexology have all been shown to help ease symptoms. Your breast care nurse or GP may be able to recommend a practitioner.
- *Antidepressants.* Low doses of antidepressants, like Citalopram and Venlafaxine, can reduce the number of flushes that you get and make them less intense. They take a couple of weeks to work, and they do have some side effects which your doctor will discuss with you.
- *Other drugs.* Gabapentin (normally given for chronic pain) and Clonidine (normally given for high blood-pressure) can also reduce the number of flushes. They take several weeks to work and also have side effects.

The National Institute for Health and Care Excellence, which provides guidance for healthcare professionals in the UK, does *not* recommend taking herbal remedies (such as black cohosh, red clover, soy products, plant oestrogens or vitamin E). This is because there is very little evidence to show that they work.

Vaginal dryness

Oestrogen is a natural vaginal lubricant. Without it, your vagina can become dry, itchy and uncomfortable, and this can make sex painful. There are several lubricants and vaginal moisturisers that can help (see page 217). If you need more than a lubricant, your oncologist may recommend a vaginal tablet (Vagifem, Ortho-Gynest) or cream (EstroGel, Ovestin). These contain a very low dose of oestrogen which is absorbed locally into the wall of the vagina. Because the amount you absorb is so small, these vaginal oestrogens are safe to use even if your cancer is sensitive to oestrogen.

Low sex drive

Women may lose interest in sex after the menopause. This can be due to physical reasons (night sweats, vaginal dryness), hormonal reasons (oestrogen boosts your sex drive) and psychological reasons (feeling less attractive after treatment). Your low sex drive can have a knock-on effect on your partner and your relationship. (For advice and tips on how to cope, see Chapter 17.)

Bladder problems

As your oestrogen levels drop, the lining of your bladder and urethra (the tube that connects your bladder to the outside world) thins and becomes more sensitive. This can lead to bladder inflammation (cystitis) where you pass urine more frequently, and urinary tract infections. You may also start to leak urine occasionally. Drinking lots of clear fluids will stop your urine from getting concentrated and dilute any bacteria. Pelvic floor exercises can also help if you start to leak urine (see page 218 for some ideas).

Tiredness and fatigue

You may feel tired, especially if your sleep is disrupted by night sweats. Severe fatigue (see pages 193–4) is uncommon but can happen. Regular exercise, like a gentle half an hour walk every day, can help give you more energy.

Weight gain

It is common to gain weight around your tummy after the menopause because your metabolism slows down. This can make it even harder to lose any extra weight you may have gained during treatment. (For advice and tips on how to cope with this, see Chapter 15.)

Mood changes

Low oestrogen levels can make you irritable and find it hard to concentrate. This can lead to mood swings, which can be unpredictable and overwhelming. Rarely, this can lead to full-blown depression. Alternatively, you may feel stressed and develop anxiety and panic attacks (see Chapter 4 for advice and help).

Skin and hair changes

Your hair can become dry and thin and your skin can feel thin, dry and itchy. Using hair conditioner and hypoallergenic soap, shower gels and moisturisers (such as baby brands) can all help. Eat a healthy, varied diet so you get enough vitamins and minerals, drink plenty of water, using a high-factor sunscreen and avoid hot showers and baths.

Every woman has to go through the menopause at some point in her life. Some women have disabling symptoms whereas others sail through, and the same can be said of treatment-induced menopause.

FERTILITY

Women are born with thousands of eggs stored in their ovaries. If you are fertile, your ovaries release an egg each month. As you get older, the number of eggs you have left gets smaller and your egg quality gets worse – both reduce your fertility. You stop producing eggs a few years before your menopause, usually in your early fifties.

As a rule of thumb, chemotherapy adds 10 years to your reproductive age, so if you're 30 when you start, you'll have the fertility of a 40-year-old when you finish. The younger you are, the more likely your fertility will return after treatment. However, if you are over 35, there is a risk that you will be infertile once your treatment finishes.

Before you start chemotherapy or have your ovaries removed, you need to think about whether you would like children in the future. This is regardless of whether you are in a relationship with someone you want to have children with, in an early or casual relationship, or single.

Questions to ask about fertility

Here are some questions you might want to ask:

- Am I fertile now?
- Will chemotherapy make me infertile?
- Can I preserve my eggs?
- Will fertility treatment delay my cancer treatment?
- Will delaying my cancer treatment to preserve my fertility make me more likely to have a recurrence or to die from my cancer?
- What do I do if I'm single?
- I already have children. Can I still preserve my eggs?
- Do I have to pay for fertility treatment?
- What are my chances of having a baby after treatment?

Liz didn't have children when she was diagnosed with breast cancer. She needed chemotherapy first, and fertility hadn't even crossed her mind. The first time it was mentioned was when she met her oncologist. Liz and her husband had to decide there and then that they were never going to have children. In hindsight, she wished she'd had the presence of mind to ask for a couple of minutes to have a private discussion with her husband instead of making a life-changing decision in front of her doctor.

Options for preserving fertility

'Ovarian function suppression' is the simplest option which shuts down your ovaries during chemotherapy with a monthly injection of a drug called Zoladex (see page 175). Your ovaries should start working again after chemotherapy, although do bear in mind that there's no guarantee.

For a greater chance of having a baby after treatment, you need more intensive treatment at a specialist fertility clinic who will guide you through the options below. Fertility treatments for cancer patients should be free on the NHS. In reality though, depending on where you live, your age and whether you already have children, you may need to pay for some of the treatment. All of these treatments are done before you start chemotherapy or have your ovaries removed. We discuss the two most common options below.

In vitro fertilisation (IVF)

This is the most effective way to preserve your fertility. Your ovaries are first stimulated with daily hormone injections to encourage them to produce more eggs. This increases the number of eggs that can be collected, and therefore increases the chance of a pregnancy in the future. If you are having chemotherapy before surgery, there is a risk that these additional hormones may stimulate your cancer to grow. If your cancer is triple negative, it is safe for you to have one or two cycles of IVF. If your cancer is ER-positive, you might be given tamoxifen or letrozole (see Chapter 13) to reduce the level of oestrogen in your body during stimulation. However, some fertility clinics may insist that you have surgery first because of the risk of cancer growth during fertility treatment.

Several eggs are then collected, fertilised outside your body with sperm from your partner or a sperm donor, and stored as embryos (fertilised eggs). They can be kept for up to 10 years before being implanted into your womb. If you are having

IVF before chemotherapy, it will delay chemotherapy by a few weeks.

Freezing non-fertilised eggs

If you are in a relationship and don't want to use your partner's sperm, or if you are single and don't want to use donor sperm, you can freeze your eggs after ovarian stimulation. These can also be stored for 10 years, before being thawed and fertilised with sperm. This gives you the option of fertilising your own eggs with the sperm of a new partner (perhaps someone you haven't met yet), although the pregnancy success rate is not as high as with IVF.

Getting pregnant after breast cancer

If your cancer is not sensitive to oestrogen and you are having chemotherapy or Herceptin, you have to continue using contraception until six months after you have finished treatment. By that time, the drugs will have left your system and can no longer harm an unborn baby.

If your cancer is sensitive to oestrogen, you will need to take tamoxifen for at least five years. You need to stop taking tamoxifen in order to get pregnant, and this means stopping treatment to prevent your cancer coming back. Most doctors advise waiting at least two years before taking a treatment break to try and get pregnant. You also can't breastfeed with tamoxifen, but you could bottle-feed if you wanted to restart sooner. In total, this could mean a two- to three-year gap from tamoxifen, which could increase the risk that your cancer might come back. You need to weigh up the pros of (hopefully) having a baby with the cons of stopping treatment to prevent your cancer back.

At the time of writing, there is currently a research trial called POSITIVE (Pregnancy Outcome and Safety of Interrupting Therapy for Women with Endocrine Responsive Breast Cancer) investigating the effect of this break in treatment on your overall survival from breast cancer. Early data from a previous trial suggested that having a baby after breast cancer treatment doesn't increase the risk of your cancer coming back or the risk of you dying from your breast cancer.

OTHER OPTIONS TO HAVE CHILDREN

If you can't have a baby naturally, there are other options available. These include using a donor egg (fertilised with your partner's sperm or donor sperm), surrogacy (where another woman carries your baby for you), adoption and fostering. You can find out further information about surrogacy at the Human Fertilisation and Embryology Authority website or the Surrogacy UK website. For information about adoption and fostering visit the Adoption UK or British Adoption and Fostering Academy website. (See page 276 for further details.)

Coming to terms with infertility

Realising that having breast cancer means that you can never have children of your own can be devastating, especially when the decision was taken away from you because of your cancer treatment.

If you are finding it hard to cope, your specialist nurse or GP can refer you to a counsellor. There is also support available online from specialist organisations such as the Daisy Network for women facing an early menopause. Breast Cancer Care has a free service called 'Someone Like Me' that can put you in touch with other women in your situation. They run 'Younger Women Together' events for women under 45 who have been diagnosed in the last three years that provide information and support. (See page 277 for further details.) Younger Breast Cancer Network

(YBCN) is a private Facebook group set up by young women with breast cancer. If you want to join, you simply send a private message to the group.

> Liz felt intense grief for the child she'd never have, and it took a good 12 months for those feelings to pass. There are other ways to welcome children into your life, such as volunteering at schools and after-school clubs, and you can also become the world's greatest auntie/friend. It can be hard when people only talk about their children (as it is for any woman who is childless). It's okay to speak up and ask your friends to change the topic every once in a while.

CHAPTER 17

RELATIONSHIPS AND SEX

BREAST CANCER WILL inevitably put a strain on your relationship with your partner and this may last for months or even years – but it may also bring you closer as you learn how to support each other through a very difficult time.

Cancer is very one-sided – it is all about you! You get the cards and the flowers and the presents and the sympathy and the attention, while your partner is often a silent witness in the background, picking up the pieces of the things you aren't able to do, such as housework, school runs or worrying about finances if you have to take time off from work. This can lead to resentment and guilt on both sides. Your partner may be unable to take time off work to come with you to every treatment and appointment, and this can leave them feeling sad and inadequate.

Alternatively, your partner may not seem to care that you have cancer and expect you to carry on with life as normal. They may not want to talk about cancer at all, maybe because they are scared about the future, or just cannot cope. The end result is that you push your partner away at the time you need them the most. Some women that Liz talked to said they had asked their husbands to divorce them because they felt so guilty about getting breast cancer and the effect it was having on their relationship. The husbands said 'no', thankfully, but it goes to show the irrationality of dealing with a cancer diagnosis.

We were very lucky. Our husbands Fraser and Dermot were incredibly supportive. They shared our devastation over the cancer diagnosis, cried with us and reassured us that they still loved us even if we only had one breast. They were able to come with us to most of our appointments and treatments, and we don't think we could have got through treatment without them. However, there were still lots of times when we were tired and irritable and got on each other's nerves.

There is no magic formula for getting through cancer with your relationship intact. You know far better than we do what does and doesn't work for you, but here are a few things that helped us.

Talk to each other

There's no 'right' time or place to have a conversation about cancer, and you may just blurt something out at the worst possible moment, but this is much better than keeping your feelings bottled up. Be explicit and tell your partner exactly how you are feeling, and then listen so you can hear their side of the story. You may both be feeling unsupported and fed up. Try not to do this late at night when you are both exhausted. You could both try keeping a diary about your feelings that you then share with each other, a bit like a private blog.

Date again

Do something together. It could be silly, like pretending you're on your first date. It could be simple like going for a walk or trying a yoga class together. It could be mundane like doing the food shopping. It's important to reconnect and forget about cancer for a while.

Trish and Fraser went on a 10-kilometre walk most days – sometimes at a snail's pace and sometimes broken part-way round at a nice tea shop. They often didn't say anything but just being together out of doors gave them some shared headspace.

Liz and Dermot borrowed a tandem bicycle, and did lots of dog walks by the sea side.

Stay in touch with your own friends

It's really important that you both keep seeing your own friends. It helps to get some breathing space away from each other, and you may find it easier to talk and work things through with friends instead of your partner.

Liz would often go for coffee with friends, but she made sure that Dermot's friends invited him out for a drink too so he had some 'not-cancer' time.

Use the local cancer centre

There may be a cancer centre (see page 183) near you and this can be a great source of help and support for you and your partner. They provide free coffee and magazines, and there is always someone to talk to. It may be nicer for your partner to escape there while you are having treatment.

Other support options

If your relationship seems to be full of tensions that you can't resolve, you could try counselling. Your doctor or GP may be able to arrange this on the NHS for free. Support groups – either face-to-face or online – may also help (see Chapter 14). If either of you think that the other is becoming anxious or depressed, you may need to encourage them to see their GP for some extra help.

Plan an end-of-treatment treat

Breast cancer treatment means putting your life on hold, and this can mean cancelling parties and holidays. If you have primary cancer, you could put something in the diary to look forward to when you've finished treatment. Plan a short break or a week away between surgery/chemotherapy and radiotherapy, and plan a longer holiday once all your hospital treatment has finished. Liz had a quick week in the sun between chemotherapy and surgery which was great to recharge. If you have secondary cancer it is more difficult because treatment never finishes, but you could still try to plan days or trips away between each treatment. Having something to look forward to is a huge psychological boost, and gives you a little dose of normality.

Breast cancer and dating

If you are single when you are diagnosed, it can be incredibly daunting to think about dating again. How will you meet someone? When do you tell them that you have cancer? When do you tell them your breasts aren't real? The Breast Cancer Care website has a great article about dating after cancer, featuring the stories of seven women in their thirties, forties and fifties. And for a brilliant, funny account of how a single woman managed the ups and downs of breast cancer without an ongoing relationship, read Anne Gildea's *I've Got Cancer, What's Your Excuse?* (Hachette Books, 2013).

TRAVEL INSURANCE

Once you have had a cancer diagnosis, travel insurance is more expensive. If you don't tell the insurance company that you have breast cancer, they will not cover you for any claim related to your cancer.

If you are planning a trip soon after you have finished surgery, chemotherapy or radiotherapy, the premiums may be even higher because the chance of you having a complication is higher at that time. Some companies will pay for your medical costs abroad, but may not automatically pay to fly you home if you need to. This option can be added as an additional cost, and you might want to consider it if you are flying in the first few weeks after finishing chemotherapy, because of the risk of a serious infection while your immune system is still low. If you have secondary cancer and are having ongoing treatment, it may be even more expensive to get insurance, but travelling abroad without adequate insurance could prove even more expensive.

Three of the most popular insurance companies that specialise in covering cancer patients are Insurancewith, Free Spirit, and World First, but others are available. You can get advice from other patients on the Macmillan and Breast Cancer Care forums. Ring several companies to get quotes for comparison and make sure you have all the details of your treatments to hand: exactly what surgery you had, which chemotherapy drugs you were given, which drugs you were taking, and the dates when everything happened. You may also need a letter from your doctor confirming that you are not travelling against medical advice.

SEX

Whether you are young or old, gay or straight, in a long-term partnership or a more casual relationship, getting breast cancer will almost certainly affect your sex life. The menopausal side effects of treatment can make sex uncomfortable or even painful, and you may lose your sex drive completely. Your altered body image after surgery can make it difficult to get naked and feel sexy in front of your partner. The mixed-up feelings of fear, guilt, anger, frustration and resentment (why me? why her? why us?) as well as the pressure of your other commitments (to children, parents, work, etc.) also have a knock-on effect. It's hardly surprising that sex can go to the very bottom of your to-do list and becomes a source of trouble (and even conflict) between you.

A lot of people find it difficult to talk about sex with their partner, let alone their doctor, and many patients give up on sex altogether, but it doesn't have to be that way. Here are our tips:

Talk about sex

If sex has become the 'elephant in the room', talk to your partner and tell them exactly what the problem is (although ideally not before you're about to have sex). It could be that you are worried it will be painful, or that they won't find you sexy, or that you simply have no desire. Listen to your partner's concerns as well – they may be scared of hurting you, or they don't know whether they should touch your scars or avoid them altogether. You might want to try counselling to help you work through these problems.

Practice on your own

Masturbation can help you get used to feeling aroused again, especially during chemotherapy, which can dull down the sensitive zones in your clitoris or penis. You can do this by yourself or with your partner, and it may help to relax you and get you in the mood. Despite what some women were taught many years ago at school or church, there is absolutely nothing wrong or dirty about using masturbation as a means of exploring what works for you and becoming more confident about sex.

Create a 'sex bag'

Sex is likely to be less spontaneous after breast cancer treatment, especially if you have vaginal dryness. Longer foreplay is part of the answer. Another solution could be a bag of tricks by the bedside. This is what we recommend:

- *Lubricant.* It can take a long time to get aroused enough to have sex, and even then, you may need additional lubricant because you are too dry. We recommend the 'YES' range of lubricants and internal moisturisers, that are also recommended by cancer nurses. They are water-based, additive-free and available on prescription and to buy online. You could also try a silicone-based lubricant, but try to use one without added chemicals.
- *Dilators.* These are good to help relax and stretch your vagina before you have sex. You can buy them online from websites such as Stress No More (see page 281 for details). Use them with lubricants during foreplay.
- *Vibrators.* You can buy small vibrators that you can use internally or externally to help you have an orgasm. You may want to try masturbating with a vibrator and dilators first, before going on to make love with your partner.

Pelvic floor muscle exercises

These exercises strengthen the muscles of your pelvic floor and can help improve your sexual enjoyment. Ideally, a specialist physiotherapist will tell you how to do them, and you may have been shown them if you have had children. Here is one that Trish used successfully after childbirth:

- Stand with your legs slightly apart. Now imagine there are some tiny people standing in an elevator at the opening of your vagina. Tighten your pelvic muscles to bring those tiny people vertically up several floors – and then relax slowly to bring them down to the 'ground floor' again. Repeat half a dozen times.

Medication

If you are still struggling with vaginal dryness despite using lubricants, your doctor can prescribe you a topical oestrogen cream (see page 217). If your partner is having trouble maintaining an erection, your doctor could prescribe a tablet like Viagra to help him.

Do other stuff

Remember that sex isn't compulsory and there are many ways of making love without penetration, orgasm or even genital contact. Simple hugs and kisses, or even a massage, can comfort you both and help you feel close during the physical and mental challenges of cancer. Go with the flow. And keep in mind that for most couples, things get a lot better once active cancer treatment is behind them.

Contraception during breast cancer treatment

You doctor will advise you to use contraception if you are having chemotherapy, HER2 treatment or tamoxifen because all of these drugs can harm an unborn baby. You may feel menopausal (e.g. if your periods stop) but could still be ovulating, so use contraception until your doctor has confirmed that you are menopausal with a blood test (see Chapter 16).

You usually can't use the oral contraceptive pill or implant injection because they contain oestrogen and/or progesterone which could stimulate any remaining breast cancer cells. Condoms are safe, although some partners are reluctant to use them. A cap is a good alternative, since neither you nor your partner can feel it, and you can insert it a bit before sex so your partner doesn't even need to know you're using it.

Another alternative is to have a coil (intrauterine device) fitted. This works by releasing a synthetic version of progesterone. However, because the hormone is released locally into your womb, very little of it enters your bloodstream, and there is no evidence to prove that a coil can cause breast cancer or increase the risk of recurrence. Once inside you, this will protect you from getting pregnant for three to five years (and you can have it removed before that if you're ready to try for a baby). The morning-after pill can be used in emergencies (for example, after a split or 'forgotten' condom) because it is only a single dose of hormones. Your GP or an NHS family planning clinic can give you more advice.

At the one time in your life when you need the support of your partner more than ever before, your breast cancer treatment may mean that you end up pushing them away. This is one of the really tough bits to deal with – trust us, we've been there too. We hope with the advice we've given you that you can show your partner how to support you, both in and out of the bedroom, and learn to have fun again.

CHAPTER 18

STAYING HEALTHY DURING AND AFTER TREATMENT

ONE OF THE most important things you can do when you are diagnosed with breast cancer is to look after your body. Staying active and eating a healthy diet will make you feel better, and there is now evidence to show that being overweight and not exercising can increase the risk of your cancer coming back.

The first thing to say is that you don't need to eat a special diet or take special supplements after a breast cancer diagnosis. Your cancer wasn't caused by eating a particular food, and there is no scientific evidence to prove that eating a particular food or food supplement will cure it. An overview of cancer prevention diets by the World Health Organization showed that the only dietary factors which increase your risk of developing breast cancer are being overweight (especially if you've already had your menopause) and drinking more than the recommended levels of alcohol.

All you need to do is eat a varied, balanced diet, try to cook most of your food from scratch (avoiding a lot of processed and packaged foods) and exercise regularly. You can eat a healthy diet whether you eat meat, are pescatarian, vegetarian or vegan. Your daily diet should include protein, fresh fruit and vegetables, carbohydrates, fibre and healthy fats. It is also safe to have things that aren't quite as good for you, so long as you eat these in moderation. Having cancer can be miserable so having little treats like chocolate can improve your morale and give you something to look forward to every day.

We recommend the following websites for specific scientific dietary advice:

- World Cancer Research Fund (www.wcrf-uk.org): 'Eating well during cancer'
- MSK Cancer Centre (www.mskcc.org): 'About Herbs, Botanicals & Other Products'
- Cathy Leman, dietician (www.dammadaboutbreastcancer.com)

If you need to have chemotherapy, this alters your sense of taste and your appetite. Try experimenting with different food flavours and textures to find something that you want to eat (we give more advice in Chapter 10). *The Royal Marsden Cancer Cookbook* has lots of recipes carefully developed and tested to tempt the palates of people going through chemotherapy and provide all the nutrients you need. They taste good even when you don't have cancer! You can access some of these recipes through Breast Cancer Care's website.

As we covered in Chapter 15, being overweight will increase your risk of recurrence. As you make it through the initial few months of cancer treatment and start to look forward to getting your life back, try to take back control of your diet and your weight and increase the amount of exercise you do. Cutting your portion sizes can help, and many women find slimming clubs can help keep them motivated. We know it's hard, but it is important.

Alcohol

Research has shown that drinking large quantities of alcohol, in particular binge-drinking in post-menopausal women, can increase the risk of your cancer coming back. It can also cause liver damage in the future. Guidance from the National Institute for Health and Care Excellence (NICE) recommends that you drink fewer than five units of alcohol a week. A unit is a small glass of wine, a single measure of a spirit or half a pint of beer. You may choose to cut out alcohol altogether, especially if it makes your hot flushes worse. However, if having a glass of wine or a gin and tonic is something you enjoy, it won't harm you if you do this a couple of times a week.

'CANCER DIETS'

There are often articles in the press suggesting that your cancer will be cured if you follow a special, often extreme, diet or take an expensive supplement. A woman may claim that 'cutting out dairy cured my cancer', but this is actually an *association* (she cut out dairy and her cancer hasn't come back), not a causal link (the change in diet *caused* the cancer not to come back). If you read the small print, the more likely *cause* for her cancer not coming back is the surgery she had, along with other treatments, such as radiotherapy and tamoxifen.

We understand that many people want to regain a sense of control following a cancer diagnosis. Manipulating what you eat is an easy way to do this and following a diet that you believe is healthy, detoxifying, strengthening or emotionally sustaining will help you feel more in control. When you read that cancer can come back despite modern medical treatments, you may be tempted to spend hundreds or even thousands of pounds on supplements and infusions, to give yourself every possible chance that your cancer won't return.

However, most of what is written about these extreme diets and supplements is shockingly inaccurate. There is very little scientific evidence to prove that their claims of cure actually work. Furthermore, restrictive diets (cutting whole food groups out) carry a real risk of malnutrition.

We advise you to steer clear of 'extreme' diets, and we're going to explain why. If, after reading the rest of this chapter, you want to try one of the cancer diets, please think about doing it alongside traditional medical treatment, so you get the best chance of a cure (see page 67 where we describe Dr Skyler Johnson's research on the poor outlook of people who reject standard medical treatment in favour of 'alternative' therapy). If you are having chemotherapy, tell your doctor about any supplements you plan to take, as these can interfere with the drugs and make chemo less effective.

Dr Jutta Huebner and her colleagues in *Anticancer Research* (January 2014) evaluated over 100 scientific studies looking at diet therapies in cancer. Dr Huebner's team identified 13 different 'cancer diets', *none* of which had been shown to increase survival in any kind of cancer. Below, we describe the pros and cons of the most popular 'cancer diets'.

Low-carbohydrate diet

A low-carb diet involves reducing the amount of carbohydrate you eat relative to other kinds of food. You cut out sugary foods (including the 'hidden sugars' in sauces, soups, yoghurts, and so on) and starchy ones (potatoes, white pasta, rice, bread) and eat more protein (eggs, lean meat, lentils), fresh vegetables and fats (butter, margarine). Variants on the low-carb diet include the 'caveman' or 'paleo' diet (cutting out foods that cavemen and women wouldn't have had access to, such as cereals) and the 'Atkins' diet.

A low-carb diet is generally pretty healthy. A lot of people eat too much white bread and refined, sugary foods, with very little fruit and veg. This diet may reduce your risk of developing type 2 diabetes and also help with weight loss (see Chapter 15), but only if your total energy intake is low, so watch your portion size too. If you're struggling with post-menopausal weight problems, cutting out carbs from your evening meal and replacing them with vegetables can be a good strategy.

Contrary to some claims, a low-carb diet does *not* work by 'starving cancer cells of sugar'. Cancer cells use sugar (glucose) as a fuel – but so do normal cells. Fast-growing cancer cells burn more sugar than slow-growing ones, just as a child who's going through a growth spurt eats more. If you don't eat any sugar or starch (which breaks down to sugar), your cancer cells *and* your normal cells will switch to burning fat or protein for fuel.

Fasting, severe calorie restriction and ketogenic diets

When you don't eat for a long period of time (for example when fasting – or indeed, during severe vomiting), your body burns its stores of fat and protein and produces a by-product called 'ketones'. A 'ketogenic diet' is another word for a diet that is so low in calories that you are effectively starving when on it. One variant of this approach is the '5+2' diet in which you eat normally (say 1,800 calories per day) for five days of every week, but on the other two days you follow a very calorie-restricted diet (usually around 600 calories).

An update focusing just on ketogenic diets was recently published in *Medical Oncology* (2017; 34: 72). It found that there is no scientific evidence that fasting boosts the immune system, clears toxins from your body or makes your cancer cells go to sleep. But there is certainly evidence that starving yourself will make you ill. You will get headaches, tiredness, muscle weakness and anaemia, and you could become so bad-tempered you'll be impossible to live with. It is also likely to take you longer to recover from breast cancer treatment because your body is weakened.

Laboratory research (either on pieces of human tissue or on mice) has suggested that chemotherapy agents work better on cells that are being 'starved'. The rationale is that these rapidly growing cells are even more likely to die during chemo if they aren't getting enough nutrients, compared to cancer cells with plenty of nutrients. At the time of writing, there is no direct evidence from *human* studies to support severe calorie restriction during cancer treatment.

However, scientists are now starting to investigate the effects of a controlled fast before chemotherapy, and there are several ongoing trials of intermittent fasting or calorie restriction during treatment for different cancers, all of which will be reporting over the next couple of years.

Macrobiotic and vegan diets

The macrobiotic diet was developed in the 1920s by a Japanese philosopher called George Ohsawa who believed that by eating a simple, healthy diet, free of toxins, it was possible to live in harmony with nature (balancing 'ying' and 'yang'). The diet is made up of organic whole grains, such as brown rice, barley and oats (comprising 50 per cent of food intake), organic fruits and vegetables (25 per cent), and soups made with vegetables, seaweed, beans, chickpeas, lentils and miso (25 per cent). Many people seeking a macrobiotic cure choose to follow a completely vegan diet with no dairy products or meats. Some people allow themselves small amounts of organic fish and meat. Nuts and seeds are encouraged; caffeine and additives are not allowed.

Although Ohsawa and others believe that a macrobiotic diet can cure cancer, there is no scientific evidence to support this claim. Furthermore, narrowing your diet to strict veganism when you're not used to doing so could make you deficient in key nutrients such as calcium, vitamin B12 and iron. There is also the risk that the very high proportion of carbohydrates in the diet may make you gain weight and/or predispose you to type 2 diabetes in the future. If you must follow a macrobiotic diet (and we don't advise it), add generous amounts of protein and include as wide a variety of different foods as you can.

Raw food diet

As you might expect, the raw food diet means eating only uncooked and unprocessed food that is also organic (hence, chemical- and preservative-free). It generally consists of an extreme vegan diet of only fruit, nuts and vegetables, though some people include raw eggs and other dairy products. It is promoted on the incorrect assumption that cooked food causes cancer and that raw food cures it. Nothing could be further from the truth.

Turmeric diet

Turmeric, a yellow spice used in curry, contains the chemical 'curcumin' which has powerful anti-inflammatory properties. Inflammation is one of the processes that leads to cancer, so curcumin is considered by some to be a possible cure. There are many websites that claim (wrongly, we believe) that turmeric helps the body destroy cancer cells, prevents the development and spread of cancer, and even makes cancer cells commit suicide. When we looked for scientific evidence on this topic, we found a lot of poor-quality studies but only four high-quality ones, of which one was in breast cancer. None demonstrated convincingly that either turmeric or curcumin improved cancer survival. The breast cancer study, published in 2010, was very preliminary and was designed to calculate the maximum tolerated dose of curcumin which would then be tested in a clinical trial. The paper stated in 2010 that a much larger trial was ongoing – but eight years later, that second (definitive) study has never been published.

Antioxidant diet

An antioxidant diet is one that aims to get rid of free radicals (highly reactive chemicals that have the potential to harm cells). A free radical gets created when an atom or a molecule either gains or loses an electron (a small negatively charged particle), causing it to become either negatively or positively charged respectively. Free radicals are formed naturally in the body in a number of key chemical reactions, but too many of them are bad for you and they may play a role in the development of cancer by damaging your genetic material. Most free radicals in the body contain oxygen (but not in a form that's good for you), and antioxidants are chemicals that neutralise free radicals (by providing the positive or negative charge to balance them).

Antioxidants in the diet include beta-carotene (an orange substance found in carrots and spinach), lycopene (a red substance found in tomatoes), vitamin A (found in mangoes, carrots, spinach, oily fish and liver), vitamin C (found in very fresh fruit and vegetables but destroyed by cooking) and vitamin E (also known as 'alpha-tocopherol' – found in seeds, nuts, leafy vegetables and vegetable oils). Most research into antioxidants uses tablets containing these vitamins.

Despite the superficial plausibility of the argument that antioxidants will reduce free radicals in the body and hence reduce the risk of developing cancer, there is no evidence that this is actually the case. Indeed, several large trials, in which half the people took antioxidant supplements and half didn't, showed no effect whatsoever. For people who already have cancer, fewer scientific studies have been done but the ones published to date suggest no benefit and even the possibility of harm (since antioxidants may *protect* cancer cells against damage from radiotherapy or chemotherapy).

Alkaline diet

Some 'cancer cure' websites (which we do not endorse) argue that cancer cells thrive in acidic conditions (low pH), so the premise is that a diet high in alkaline foods will help fight cancer. 'Alkaline' foods are said to include fruit, nuts, legumes and vegetables. 'Neutral' ones are said to include natural fats, starch and sugar. 'Acidic' foods are described as including meat, fish, dairy products, eggs, grains and alcohol.

The alkaline diet for cancer is a complete myth. The pH of your body is tightly controlled by enzymes, and is only altered when you are seriously ill, for example a life-threatening infection or a heart attack. Your body's acidity cannot be altered by changing your diet. All the food you eat, whether it is acidic or alkaline, is neutralised by enzymes in your gut when you digest it.

The idea that alkaline diets cure cancer simply does not make biological sense. Whilst some cancer cells do have a tendency to generate a slightly more acidic environment than non-cancer cells, due to differences in how they use nutrients and generate energy, no cell (cancerous or otherwise) can survive in a purely alkaline environment. Despite a lot of speculation in the non-scientific literature, there is absolutely no evidence that changing the acidity of a person's diet will lead to any change whatsoever in the acidity of their body, nor is there any evidence that doing so will change the outcome of cancer.

'Named' anti-cancer diets

You may come across 'cancer diets' named after their founders, for example:

- *Gerson's regimen*: claims to stimulate your metabolism and reduce bodily toxins using extracts of raw liver, pancreas, thyroid and iodine. Despite a book claiming scientific proof, an enthusiastic website and a Gerson Research Organization, this regimen isn't backed up by scientific research and it doesn't cure cancer.
- *Gonzalez regimen*: a similar rationale to Gerson but recommends freeze-dried pancreatic enzymes, coffee enemas and high-dose vitamins. Again, this is not evidence-based.
- *Breuss cure*: involves living on nothing but vegetable juice, fruit juice and herbal tea for six weeks with the aim of 'starving the tumour'. A well-described side effect is malnutrition and it is conceivable that you could starve yourself to death. Don't try it.
- *Budwig diet*: requires you to eat little more than omega-3 fatty acids (such as flaxseed oil) and proteins with high sulphur content (things like curd cheese), on the flawed assumption that cancer arises from too many trans fats and not enough omega-3s and that reversing this balance will cure cancer. Budwig is said to have sold a lot of curd cheese but there's no evidence that this has ever cured any cancers.

We hope that the above list warns you off jumping on the cancer diet bandwagon. We also caution strongly against taking high-dose vitamins or folic acid because, in theory at least, fast-growing cancer cells may be stimulated by these micronutrients.

If your oncologist has suggested taking a particular vitamin or mineral (for example, iron to correct anaemia or a calcium and vitamin D complex to strengthen your bones) follow his or her advice at the dose they recommend. Don't fall into the trap of thinking that the more mega-vitamins you take, the better your chance of a cure.

In conclusion, extreme diets won't cure your cancer – but surgery, radiotherapy and chemotherapy might.

EXERCISE

There are three main reasons why you should exercise after a breast cancer diagnosis. First, regular physical activity has been shown to reduce the risk of recurrence, and exercise is now recommended in the NICE guidelines for treating breast cancer.

Second, exercise during and after cancer treatment can reduce fatigue, improve your sense of well-being and quality of life, and also help to prevent weight gain, which also reduces your risk of recurrence. Being inactive rarely helped anyone get better from any disease. Physical inactivity, especially lying in bed, can lead to blood clots in your legs, and your risk of clotting is higher after a cancer diagnosis. It also leads to fatigue, muscular deconditioning and loss of heart fitness. The most common cause of death in women who have had breast cancer is heart disease. Doing half an hour of moderate exercise every day (that is, exercise that makes you a bit out of breath and makes you sweat but doesn't make you gasp) can help strengthen your heart, especially if you have had chemotherapy or Herceptin treatment that can weaken it.

Third, exercise can help improve the side effects of breast cancer treatment. Walking every day during chemotherapy has been shown to reduce the side effects of chemo. We were both told by other patients to walk for half an hour every day, even if we felt absolutely rotten and could only go to the end of the road and back. We're certain we felt better for it, and encourage you to do the same. Exercise, such as swimming, can also help with lymphoedema (see page 96). Finally, if you are taking an Aromatase Inhibitor to prevent recurrence (see page 172), your bones will have a tendency to thin. Regular weight-bearing exercise, such as jogging, tennis and aerobics, will help strengthen your bones.

Broadly speaking, there are three different kinds of exercise:

1. *Aerobic exercise* (such as aerobics and cycling) which builds cardiovascular fitness by increasing your heart rate, working your muscles and making you breathe faster.
2. *Strengthening (or resistance) exercise* which focuses on muscle-building through weights or holding postures (such as squats, lunges and using dumbbells).
3. *Flexibility exercise* (such as yoga and Pilates) which involves stretching to increase suppleness.

To get the most benefit, you should do something that is weight-bearing, that gets you breathing hard and builds up a sweat. Ideally you should do a minimum of 30 minutes' moderate exercise five times a week, with a mixture of aerobic and strength-training exercise. Slowly, your fitness levels will return, and you may even get fitter than before, once you appreciate your body and everything it has coped with so far.

If you exercised before breast cancer, try to go back to it after treatment. You'll be advised not to do anything strenuous for the first few weeks after your operation to let everything heal (although you should still walk every day), and your surgeon will tell you when they are happy for you to start exercising properly again. You may need to ease back into sports such as swimming, tennis and yoga as your arm mobility improves.

Our advice is: do something you enjoy and do it often. Here are some additional tips:

- *Use your common sense.* If an exercise programme doesn't feel right, don't follow it just because you've heard that others are doing it. You may have other conditions (e.g. osteoporosis, diabetes, sciatica), so you need to take account of all of them.

- *Listen to your doctors.* If you're at all concerned, ask them if it's okay to start exercising again, and if there is anything you shouldn't do. If you are otherwise healthy, you can return to just about any sport once your wounds are healed, even rock climbing.
- *Start slowly and work up.* Even if you were pretty fit before your diagnosis of breast cancer, surgery, radiotherapy, chemotherapy and Herceptin all take their toll on the body. You may find that when you do start exercising again you can barely make it round the block! Don't worry – this is normal. Give yourself a break, forget what you used to be able to do and don't compare yourself to anyone else. Set modest, achievable goals – little and often is the key.
- *Warm up before exercising.* The older you get, the longer you need to warm up before a workout, and this is doubly true if you are feeling tired and sluggish after all your treatment. Don't set off at a sprint and pull your hamstring! Start with a gentle jog.
- *Listen to your body.* Stop exercising if you feel pain or something feels wrong. Rest is just as important to let your body heal, especially if you are having chemotherapy. We found during chemo that the first few minutes of a walk were the worst (feeling sick, exhausted, even having to stop to breathe and spit) but things usually got better as we carried on. On your very worst days it may be better to call it a day and get back on the sofa.
- *Join a class.* A recent review article in the *British Journal of Sports Medicine* (September 2017) showed that cancer patients are more likely to gain physical and psychological benefit from exercise if they join a class – mostly because the class motivates them to turn up! A class can also be a good way to meet new people. There should be special exercise and swimming classes for cancer patients in your area, and your cancer nurse will be able to give you more information. If you go to a 'regular' class, let the instructor know that you that you are having (or have recently had) cancer

treatment, so they can give you extra help and support, if needed.

- *Use an app.* If you're the sort of person who organises your life on your smartphone, there are numerous apps available offering training videos and customisable programmes, such as the 'Couch to 5k' programme.
- *Set yourself a target.* Macmillan, Breast Cancer Care and Breast Cancer Now, as well as smaller cancer charities, organise sponsored walks, swims, bike rides, triathlons and treks in the UK and abroad to raise money. They can be great fun and highly motivating. Have a browse on the websites of the main cancer charities to find something that takes your fancy. This is a great way of giving something back through fundraising, and your family and friends may want to join in as well.

We were both active before we were diagnosed, and managed to exercise during chemotherapy. Liz did a very slow sprint-distance triathlon halfway through. Trish power-walked 10k most days. However, we learned not to compare our chemo performance to what we used to do. Towards the end of chemo, we became more and more tired, and did less and less – often just a (short) daily walk, or a jog in our good weeks. However, after a few months, our fitness slowly came back. Within a year we joined the all-night women-only 100km bike ride 'Ride the Night' to raise money for female cancer charities.

If you want more detail on the benefits of physical activity and breast cancer, the Macmillan website has some excellent resources (see page 28 for details). There's also a useful post-cancer workout book called *The Breast Cancer Survivor's Fitness Plan* (McGraw-Hill 2006).

Walking

Walking is the most common form of exercise that most women do during and after breast cancer, and it's free. All you need is a decent pair of trainers. You can do it alone, maybe listening to a podcast or an audiobook, or walk with a friend and have a gossip at the same time. If you've never walked before, try these suggestions for 'walking workouts':

- *Slow-fast-medium (about 30 minutes)*: Walk gently to warm up for 5 minutes, then walk as fast as you can for 10 minutes. Remember where you got to, then turn around and walk back briskly, gradually slowing down to cool down as you get closer to home. If 30 minutes is too much, just do 5 minutes' fast walking before turning around. See if you can walk further every time.
- *Mindfulness walk (about 30 minutes)*: Go for a walk near a river, in a park or by the sea – somewhere beautiful and inspiring to look at. As you walk, feel each step – first the heel strike, then the foot roll, then the lift-off of your toes. Breathe slowly and deeply and notice things you find beautiful, curious or symbolic (an unusual wild flower, the cockerel on a church spire, three buses in a row). Be aware of your body moving through space; be conscious of your breathing, and of the sun, wind or rain on your face.
- *Slow talk-walk (1–2 hours)*: When someone suggests they pop by to visit you, suggest you go for a walk instead of (or as well as) having coffee or lunch. Choose your café, and work out a nice route to it. Because this is a longer walk, it doesn't have to be fast or make you breathless. If the weather is nice, pack a lovely picnic instead.
- *Nordic walking (1–2 hours)*: This is a great form of exercise with special walking poles. The poles are designed to take some of your body weight off your hips and knees, and your arms and shoulders also get a workout. They are great when walking in the countryside, especially if it is hilly. Just search

for 'Nordic walking poles' on the Internet for classes and suppliers near you.

- *Walk-run.* If you want to learn to run, or used to run before getting cancer, the free NHS 'Couch to 5k' app is great to get you running again. It's aimed at beginners, and, over nine weeks, you progress from walking with a little bit of jogging, to running for 30 minutes or 5km without stopping. You can repeat each week if nine weeks is too much for you.

Swimming

Swimming and aqua-aerobics classes are great options after breast surgery because they strengthen your back, shoulder and tummy muscles as well as your heart. Check with your surgeon and make sure they are happy for you to start swimming after your operation. If you have had a mastectomy, you can buy a mastectomy swimsuit with a pocket for your prosthesis (order a free aqua prosthesis from Knitted Knockers UK – www.kkukciowix.com). Some pools may offer swimming lessons and ladies-only sessions if you are self-conscious about your appearance.

What you do in the water will depend on how strong a swimmer you were before you got cancer. Even if you've never swum before, you can gain a lot of strength, fitness and flexibility from a regular session in the pool. Make sure that you warm up and cool down with a couple of slow, gentle lengths every time.

Here are some ideas:

- *Walk up and down the pool.* Water provides both support and resistance, so it's great for exercising even if you aren't actually swimming. You need a pool that doesn't get too deep and isn't too crowded. You could ask at the reception desk when the quietest times to swim are. Walk in long big strides from one end of the pool to the other, taking your time and using the lane ropes for support if you need them. Rest until you're recovered, then repeat. This is an excellent exercise if you're overweight and/or have bad hips or knees that prevent you from walking far on dry land.

- *Slow lap swimming for 30 minutes.* Try swimming one length in your favourite stroke, and then swim back using another stroke. Don't go too fast, and stop to rest at the end of each lap if you need to. Swimming can be tiring, and it does take time to build up your fitness.

- *Kicking.* If you already swim well, try using a polystyrene kick-board for a few lengths in between your normal laps. You can often use them for free in many public pools. Hold the kick-board in front of you with both hands, push off the wall and kick (either front crawl or breast-stroke legs). This is hard work and you may feel like you are going backwards at times. Practice makes perfect!

- *Fast repeats.* Once you have warmed up with four to eight lengths, try swimming two lengths as fast as you can, and then stop for as long as you need to get your breath back. Repeat five times. These shorter, faster bursts will really help build your fitness.

Cycling

Even if you've never ridden a bike before, or it's been a long time, it can be a great way to get fit and meet other people. We recommend the British Cycling Breeze rides for women and led by women, to get women into cycling. There are also lots of cycling clubs all over the UK who have rides for beginners. You don't need a new shiny bike or expensive Lycra kit, just a bike that is roadworthy, a helmet and a puncture kit, some comfortable sports gear and trainers. If you have an exercise bike at home, you could use that to get fit instead.

Here are some ideas:

- *Exercise bike (20–30 minutes).* Riding a bike inside can be boring. We both either listen to music, or watch box sets on the TV or a tablet while cycling. Pedal gently for 5 minutes to warm up, and increase the pace or resistance for 5–10 minutes – you should be breathing fast but still able to carry on a conversation, before you then cool down. Start pedalling for 10 minutes and see how you feel. Try increasing your time by one minute every day and/or upping the resistance a bit.

- *Road bike 10-mile loop (about an hour).* Make sure your bike is roadworthy, you're wearing a helmet, your tyres are pumped and you have a phone, some money and a puncture repair kit. You could just leave the house for a gentle ride and turn around after half an hour, or look at a map and plan a 10–12-mile route. Go slowly at first, and have fun! You may want to take a bottle of water and snack with you (raisins or chocolate) to keep you going. As you gain in confidence and fitness, increase your distance and pace.
- *Road bike weekend ride (2–3 hours on the bike, plus social time).* When you've regained your confidence on the bike with a few short rides, why not make a social event of it? Round up some family or friends, and plan a ride out to your favourite café or lunch stop. Eating cake is a very important part of social cycling – and you've earned it!

Yoga

Yoga is sometimes described as a way of life. Originating in India, it includes physical, mental and spiritual elements in the form of physical exercises (to increase strength, flexibility and breathing), relaxation and mindfulness (see Chapter 14). There is a lot of research that shows yoga can improve fatigue, anxiety, depression, stress levels, sleep quality and overall quality of life for breast cancer patients.

There are many different kinds of yoga, and some are more vigorous than others. Active yoga focuses more on strength and flexibility, while restorative yoga focuses on relaxation and mindfulness. If you have never done yoga before, you should try to go to a class first so the teacher can show you how to get into and out of poses, make sure you are in the right position, and that you know how to breathe properly as you move between the poses. You will also get to meet new people too. Tell the instructor which treatments you have had, so they can make adjustments for any difficult poses. Most yoga centres will let you hire mats.

After this, you can do yoga at home with a book, DVD or app to guide you. If you're stiff and have never done yoga before, try *Yoga for the Stiffer Body* by Lin Craddock and colleagues (My Yoga Tutor, 2016, available on Kindle only). If you want a yoga book that is directed at people with breast cancer, try Dr Jimmy Kwok's *Yoga for Breast Cancer Survivors and Patients* (Acorn Independent Press, 2017). To get started, all you need is a non-slip surface (ideally, a yoga mat) and some light, loose clothes (e.g. a T-shirt and leggings).

Trish didn't do yoga during cancer treatment but she discovered it subsequently and now does 45 minutes every morning, using Judith Lasater's *30 Essential Yoga Poses* (Rodmell Press, 2004), which is not specifically aimed at people with cancer.

Liz did some yoga before her treatment. She goes to aerial yoga classes (where your body weight is supported by a hammock, which is good if you have stiff or weak shoulders after surgery) and uses the Cody app at home.

Other activities

As we said earlier, there is no 'best' physical activity for helping you through breast cancer. Do what you love, even if nobody else you know is doing it! As long as it gets your heart pumping and it makes you feel good, it will help. Whether it's tennis, rock climbing or Zumba, or something less strenuous like Pilates or tai chi, whether you start playing hockey or netball again or take up a completely new sport, have fun.

Advice for sporty people with breast cancer

There is very little research on exercise for people who regularly exercise, train and race who are having cancer treatment, and very few doctors are taught how to advise you. We were both very sporty before we were diagnosed and we got most of our advice about exercising during treatment from other sporty patients. We want to share what we've learned.

It is usually safe to carry on training during your breast cancer treatment, apart from when you are recovering from surgery (your doctor will tell you when you can start training again). However, in the beginning you will not be able to train as hard or as long as you used to. This is because chemotherapy lowers your immunity and affects your heart, radiotherapy can be exhausting and Herceptin also has potentially damaging effects on the heart. If you try to maintain the intensity and duration of exercise you enjoyed before cancer, you may end up collapsing on the floor in a heap. The most important thing is to make sure that your body has enough energy to heal and that your immune system improves so you can recover promptly and race well in the future.

Whatever sport you do, you should dial it down during treatment. Think slow base training in a low heart rate zone or short high-intensity cardio and strength sessions as you get your energy back. Once you have finished treatment there is no reason why you can't get back to your normal training routine. Accept that returning to peak fitness will take time (probably at least a year). Don't sign up for races three months after finishing treatment and expect to put in a fast time. You may, however, want to enter an event just to complete it and show others that you can still take part despite breast cancer.

Think about adding in some strength and conditioning and flexibility sessions to give yourself some variety and help restore a general level of all-round fitness. Ask someone in the gym to help you with a bodyweight programme. Think of it as a chance to start over and train your body properly, building up from scratch. Ignore your previous personal best times and try not to compare yourself to others. You could also check out the website www.cancerfit.me which provides evidence-based exercise and training resources for people living with and beyond cancer.

Treatment affects everybody differently, regardless of their fitness. It may take months or even years to get your fitness back, but it should come back, and you may even end up going faster or farther than before!

BREAST CANCER DURING
PREGNANCY

WORLDWIDE, THREE TO eight pregnancies in every 100,000 are affected by breast cancer. To put this another way, in the UK, of the hundreds of thousands of women diagnosed each year with cancer, fewer than 100 of these women will be pregnant at the time.

It can be very challenging to detect a breast cancer during pregnancy because your breasts are constantly changing. If you are at all concerned, you should see your GP. Any area of concern will be assessed with an ultrasound. If you need a mammogram, it will be done with a protective shield on your tummy because the X-rays can harm your unborn baby. A core biopsy (see page 12) will also be taken from any suspicious areas in your breast or lymph nodes to analyse them further.

If breast cancer is found in your lymph nodes, you can't have staging CT or bone scans (which are normally done to look for distant disease – see page 28) because of the risk to the baby from the radiation dose. Instead, you may have a chest X-ray (with a tummy shield) and a liver ultrasound scan. You can have the more accurate CT and bone scans after you have given birth.

How to cope

Being pregnant is meant to be one of the most exciting times in your life. Sadly, however, this excitement can turn into despair with a cancer diagnosis. It can be hard to find help from people who know what you're going through. That's where the fabulous charity Mummy's Star can help (see page 281 for details). It focuses on supporting women and their families who are affected by a cancer diagnosis during pregnancy or within the first year of giving birth. Their website is full of information about coping with work, financial aid and benefits, maternity and sick leave, as well as offering forums for women and their partners, and advice on how to support your children. If you are diagnosed with breast cancer while you are pregnant, we urge you to go to the website for further support.

It is unlikely that you will need to end your pregnancy (a 'medical abortion') in order to treat your breast cancer. Most pregnant women are able to have some treatment, although your delivery may be earlier than planned. It is your decision, however, and you may choose to have a termination.

There is no evidence to show that having an abortion improves the prognosis of your breast cancer. This means that women who keep their baby probably have the same chance of surviving their breast cancer as those who choose to have an abortion.

Will you be able to breastfeed?

You shouldn't breastfeed during chemotherapy because the drugs can pass to your baby in your breast milk and potentially cause harm. You also shouldn't breastfeed with Herceptin for the same reason. If you don't need Herceptin, you can still continue to express milk (that you can't give to your baby) so your supply doesn't dry up. When you have finished chemotherapy, you can then breastfeed your baby.

QUESTIONS TO ASK YOUR DOCTOR

- Have you treated pregnant women with cancer before?
- How will you involve my obstetrician (the doctor looking after your pregnancy)?
- Do I need treatment right away, or can it wait until I've had my baby?
- What are the treatment options?
- Do I need to consider ending the pregnancy so I can have breast cancer treatment?
- If I delay treatment, could it affect the chance of my cancer coming back?
- How will the treatment affect me and my baby?
- Can I breastfeed?

Will your treatment be different?

Because breast cancer during pregnancy is so rare, there are no hard and fast rules for treatment. Every case is different. Your cancer will be discussed at an MDT with your oncologist and an obstetrician (a doctor who specialises in pregnancy), and your treatment will be planned to give the best possible outcome for you and your baby.

What treatment you have depends on how far along in your pregnancy you are. Pregnancy is divided into three-monthly sections called 'trimesters' (0–12 weeks; 13–28 weeks; and 29–40 weeks), and different treatment options are recommended for each one. These are the basic principles:

- *You can have surgery in any trimester.* There will be an obstetrician monitoring your baby while you are having your operation. There is a small risk of miscarriage with a general anaesthetic.

- *You can have chemotherapy in trimesters two and three* (from 13 weeks onwards) and this is the most common treatment. You can then have surgery and radiotherapy when you have delivered your baby.
- *You cannot have radiotherapy* when you are pregnant because it can harm your baby – this might affect which operation you have.
- *You cannot have Herceptin* when you are pregnant because it can harm your baby.
- *You cannot have hormone therapy* when you are pregnant because it can harm your baby.

Your medical team may discuss delivering your baby earlier than planned. They may suggest this so that you can start Herceptin treatment, for example.

Will your prognosis be worse because you're pregnant?

Getting breast cancer when you're pregnant does not mean that you have a higher chance of it coming back or dying from breast cancer when compared to a woman who isn't pregnant. However, because a lot of pregnant women are diagnosed late, often when their cancer has spread to their lymph nodes, their overall outlook is worse than a woman whose breast cancer was diagnosed at an earlier stage.

If you get breast cancer when you are pregnant, your survival and recurrence rates are the same as non-pregnant women who have the same cancer as you. While chemotherapy can affect your future fertility (see Chapter 16), the treatment you have during this pregnancy will not harm children from any future pregnancies.

CHAPTER 20

BREAST CANCER IN MEN

BREAST CANCER IN men is rare, but it does happen. Around 350 men are diagnosed with breast cancer every year in the UK (compared with over 55,000 women), and they are normally diagnosed in their sixties and over. Because male breast cancer is uncommon, less is known about it, and most of the research into treatment and survival has been carried out on women.

Why do men get breast cancer?

All men have a very small amount of breast tissue behind their nipples, which is why you can get breast cancer. Ninety per cent of male breast cancers are sensitive to oestrogen, a female sex hormone, and while you don't have ovaries, you do produce a small amount of oestrogen in your fat. Anything that increases your exposure to oestrogen, such as some prostate cancer treatments, being overweight and liver damage due to alcohol, will increase your risk of breast cancer. Exposure to environmental chemicals, such as pollutants and petroleum solvents, previous radiotherapy for Hodgkin's lymphoma and the genetic condition Klinefelter syndrome (in which men have an extra female chromosome) can also increase your risk. You may also have a mutation in the BRCA 1 or 2 genes (see page 30) that increases your lifetime risk of getting breast cancer from 0.1 per cent to 10 per cent; this kind of breast cancer is more likely if you have a strong family history of breast cancer at a young age.

Differences in how it is detected

Because your breasts are much smaller than a woman's, your symptoms are slightly different. Most men normally feel a hard lump close to the nipple. You may also notice that your nipple has been pulled in, or find a rash on your nipple (which can be mistaken for 'jogger's nipple'). Other signs are bloody nipple discharge or a lump in your armpit. If you are concerned, see your GP for an urgent check-up. Because men don't expect to get breast cancer, it tends to be more advanced by the time it is diagnosed, though this is not the case in all men.

If your GP is concerned, they will refer you to your local breast clinic where you will have the same set of tests that a woman would have (see Chapter 3). Please don't feel embarrassed about being referred to the breast clinic. The doctors and nurses are used to seeing male patients, and will do their best to make you feel at ease. It may help to take someone with you for moral support.

Differences in how it is treated

The principles of treatment are the same – namely, surgery, followed by additional treatments, such as chemotherapy, radiotherapy and hormone therapy, if needed, to reduce the chance that your cancer will come back. These are all explained in earlier chapters, which are relevant to men as well as women. However, there are a few subtle differences that we will go through below.

Surgery

Because you only have a very small amount of breast tissue, your surgeon will do a mastectomy to treat the breast cancer. This includes removing your nipple. There are options available to improve the cosmetic appearance of your chest after surgery such as lipofilling, nipple reconstruction or a nipple tattoo (see Chapter 8).

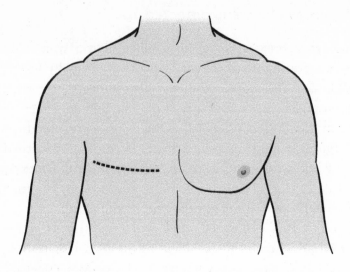

Male mastectomy scar

Hormone therapy

If your cancer is sensitive to oestrogen, you will be given a tablet called tamoxifen to stop any remaining breast cancer cells responding to oestrogen (see Chapter 10). Tamoxifen causes menopausal symptoms in women, and you may find that you have these symptoms as well (see Chapter 16).

Fertility

If you need chemotherapy, the drugs will damage your sperm cells so sperm production slows down or stops altogether. If you think you might want to have children in the future (whether it's your first or another child, or just keeping your options open if you don't have a current partner), your sperm can be collected before you start chemotherapy. The sperm is then frozen until you want to use it. This is called sperm-banking and the sperm is normally kept for 10 years. Treatment should be free on the NHS because you are having cancer treatment, but this is not always the case.

Life with male breast cancer

You may lose your sex drive (libido) during treatment for one of two reasons. The first is psychological – dealing with the mental impact of a cancer diagnosis combined with a loss of self-esteem or depression. The second reason is due to the treatments themselves, namely chemotherapy and hormone therapy, which can lower your libido and make it difficult to get an erection. Treatment may also make you simply too tired for sex.

We talk about sex and relationships in detail in Chapter 17. It's important to talk to your partner about how you are feeling. There are many ways of making love without having penetrative sex, and it can help to maintain some degree of intimacy during this emotionally challenging time. If you are finding it difficult to maintain an erection sufficient to achieve penetration, your GP may be able to prescribe you a drug such as Viagra (though some other medical conditions mean that Viagra is not an option for all men).

Where you can find support

Because breast cancer in men is so rare, you may feel very alone. It may be frustrating that all the information you find online is directed at women, and that the media associate the colour pink with breast cancer, forgetting that men get breast cancer too. The UK charity Breast Cancer Care has an excellent leaflet available on their website called 'Men With Breast Cancer', and we encourage you to read it. Your breast care nurse and GP are a good source of support, and you may also want to try their online forum (see page 277) for men with breast cancer. This is where you'll find other men who have had breast cancer and their stories may help you get your head round what's happening to *you*.

BREAST CANCER IN LGBT+ PEOPLE

THERE IS VERY little specific research on breast cancer in people who identify as lesbian, bisexual, gay, trans, intersex, queer and other sexual orientations (which we'll abbreviate as 'LGBT+'). This is mainly because cancer registries (the big databases that hold details of everyone with cancer in the UK, unless they've asked for their details to be withheld) do not routinely record details of people's sexual orientation. Some LGBT+ pressure groups are campaigning for such data to be collected so that any inequalities of provision and differences in outcome can be highlighted. At the moment, however, the evidence base on this subject is very limited – so please read this chapter with that in mind.

Being lesbian, gay or bisexual doesn't appear to increase your risk of getting breast cancer – but it doesn't decrease that risk either. Since breast cancer is *very* common in women, many women who get it are lesbian or bisexual. Breast cancer is rare in men but it happens, and some of those men will be gay. For the general risk factors for breast cancer (and hence an answer to the question 'why me?'), see Chapter 1 for women and Chapter 20 for men.

Statistically speaking, lesbians are slightly more likely than straight women to be overweight and to drink more than the recommended levels of alcohol – both of which increase the risk of breast cancer. They are also more likely to have never had children (another risk factor).

If you are a gay man (and not trans), your risk of breast cancer and how it is likely to affect you appears to be very similar to how it affects any man (see Chapter 20).

If you are transsexual – either female to male or male to female, and at any stage in your transition – there is very little published research. We found only two major studies. One – by Louis Gooren's team in the *Journal of Sexual Medicine* (December 2013) – was from the Netherlands. These researchers collected data on 2,307 male-to-female and 795 female-to-male transsexuals who had been exposed to cross-sex hormones (that is, oestrogens in the former and androgens in the latter) for between 5 and 30 years. Reassuringly, they found only one proven case (and another possible case) of breast cancer in male-to-female transsexuals and one case in the female-to-male transsexuals. The second study – by Brown and Jones in *Breast Cancer Research and Treatment* (November 2014) – was of 5,135 transgender US veterans; 10 cases of breast cancer were detected: 7 in male-to-female and 3 in female-to-male transsexuals.

The absolute numbers of breast cancers found in these studies are small but they are consistent with the conclusion that the risk of developing breast cancer in both trans men and trans women is approximately the same as it is in cis men – and a lot less than it is in cis women.

LGBT+ people and the healthcare system

In surveys, a minority of LGBT+ people have felt that health professionals caring for them have sometimes 'treated me differently', 'refused to care for me', 'blamed me for my condition' or 'used excessive precautions'. Worrying (consciously or subconsciously) whether we're going to encounter this kind of behaviour in health professionals would make most of us reluctant to come forward. Research has shown that lesbian and trans people are less likely to attend for breast screening, so breast cancer *may* be less likely to be picked up early. And for the same reasons, some LGBT+ people (though by no means all) may feel less comfortable attending a health check-up or seeing their GP with symptoms that could be breast cancer.

Some blogs by LGBT+ people with cancer have commented on 'heteronormative' and 'cis-normative' assumptions made by healthcare staff. A woman's lesbian partner, for example, may be treated as her 'friend' or 'sister' by staff who assume that her husband is at work. This can be particularly upsetting when you're in a vulnerable state waiting for cancer test results or a dose of chemotherapy. You will need to play it by ear, but as a general rule we recommend that you introduce your partner as your partner, explain that s/he is a partner, not just a friend, and (if this is your wish) that you'd like her/him involved in your decision-making discussions. But we're aware that the power dynamics and attitudes of staff may not always be conducive to open and honest dialogue. We hope that most – and ideally all – of your encounters with healthcare staff are supportive and non-judgemental (doctors and nurses are certainly expected to be open and accepting as part of their job).

The bottom line is: breast cancer is no respecter of sexual orientation. Whether you identify as gay, straight, bi, trans, intersex or queer, follow the general advice in this book and elsewhere for having breast screening, seeking prompt advice on breast symptoms and asking for help (if you need it) in making your choices about treatment. Try to identify a health professional you feel comfortable with and (to the extent that you trust them) be honest with them about your concerns about your wider care.

Where you can find support

You may find it incredibly isolating having breast cancer as an LGBT+ person. Most cancer charities include sections on their websites for LGBT+ people and, of course, all the information and general support is relevant to everyone. Macmillan, for example, has a downloadable booklet on LGBT people with cancer (www.macmillan.org.uk/_images/lgbt-people-with-cancer_tcm9-282785.pdf), as do Breast Cancer Care (www.breastcancercare.org.uk/sites/default/files/files/lesbian_and_bisexual_women_and_breast_cancer_report.pdf) and Living Beyond Breast Cancer (www.lbbc.org/get-support/print/guides-to-understanding/breast-cancer-infocus-getting-care-you-need-lesbian-gay-or).

Breast Cancer Care and Macmillan may have forum entries for LGBT+ people, but there is a chance that they won't be active when you need them. There are a few specific LGBT+ websites that you might want to look at to get immediate support for you and your loved ones. In the UK, both the National LGBT Cancer Project (https://lgbtcancer.org/about/) and the LGBT Foundation (www.lbbc.org/lgbt-breast-cancer/your-medical-needs/disparities-breast-cancer-risk-and-care-lesbian-gay-and) offer support and advice for LGBT+ people with cancer. In the US, the National LGBT Cancer Project (https://lgbtcancer.org) provides support, services and research for LGBT+ cancer patients.

CHAPTER 22

BREAST CANCER IN OLDER PEOPLE

AN OLDER PERSON used to be defined as anyone over the age of 65, but because people are living longer and are generally healthier than in the past, doctors now tend to divide patients into the under-seventies and over-seventies.

Age, however is just a number. You may feel old before you turn 70, and likewise you may still feel young in your eighties. Although the principles of treating breast cancer are the same if you are over 70, your doctor does need to take into account how mentally and physically fit you are before they plan your treatment.

Age differences in screening for breast cancer

In the UK, women are offered a breast screening mammogram every three years between the ages of 50 and 70, with the aim of identifying small breast cancers at an early stage. If you are older than 70 and haven't yet had breast cancer, there is still a chance that you might develop it in the future. This is because the biggest risk factor for getting breast cancer is getting older, so your risk increases with age. A third of all breast cancers are diagnosed in the over-seventies (around 13,000 women a year). If you are over 70 and you would like to continue to be screened for breast cancer, you can self-refer for an NHS mammogram every three years by contacting your local breast screening unit (or ask your GP).

As with younger women, if you develop symptoms that might be caused by breast cancer (especially a new lump in the breast), see your GP promptly whether or not you have had a screening mammogram in the past.

Age differences in how breast cancer is detected

Older women are more likely to notice a lump or a change in their breast compared to women in their fifties and sixties who are more likely to be diagnosed through screening. Breast cancer in older women is generally slow-growing, sensitive to oestrogen, with a relatively good prognosis. However, because many older women stop checking their breasts and no longer have regular mammograms, their cancer may not be diagnosed until it is at a later stage and has already spread to the lymph nodes. This means that they need more intensive treatment compared to women with cancers picked up at an earlier stage, and they may or may not be fit enough to cope with these treatments.

Age differences in how breast cancer is treated

The basic principles of diagnosing, staging and treating breast cancer are the same in people of all ages – and hence, all the other sections of this book apply equally to people over 70 and under 70.

The mainstay of treatment is still surgery, and this will either be a lumpectomy followed by radiotherapy, or a mastectomy (see Chapter 7). It is much more difficult to reshape or reconstruct an older woman's breast because of the effects of ageing on the breast skin and tissue. Before you have an operation, you need to be checked to see if you are fit enough to withstand the physical stress of an operation and an anaesthetic. Things that may affect this are heart, lung and kidney problems, such as high blood pressure and a previous stroke or heart attack. If your doctor doesn't think you are well enough to have a general anaesthetic, they may be able to operate using a local anaesthetic and some sedation (which makes you drowsy and often stops you remembering what happened afterwards). If this is thought to be too much for you, and your cancer is sensitive to oestrogen, you may be able to have hormone therapy instead of an operation (see Chapter 13).

If you have a cancer with a poor prognosis or your cancer is not sensitive to oestrogen, your doctor may need to discuss chemotherapy or Herceptin therapy with you (see Chapters 10 and 11). A lot of older people have chemotherapy for blood cancers like leukaemia and lymphoma, and being old does not mean that you can't or shouldn't have treatment. However, your doctor needs to make sure that you are fit enough to cope with chemotherapy or Herceptin, and that you are likely to live long enough to see the benefits from these treatments.

Older people are less likely to be included in research trials of chemotherapy, but there are also trials looking at the benefits of radiotherapy in older women, and your doctor will talk to you about these if they are involved in the trials.

QUESTIONS TO ASK YOUR DOCTOR

It is important to have a full and frank conversation with your doctors about what is right for *you*. The following questions may help:

- What treatment would you offer someone with my kind of breast cancer who was in their fifties?
- How will my other medical problems affect my breast cancer treatment? Could the treatment make them worse?
- What happens if I don't have any treatment?
- How will my treatment affect my quality and length of life?
- If I don't an operation, how will you monitor my cancer to see if it's growing?
- Do I need to have radiotherapy? Are there any radiotherapy trials I could go into?
- If I was fitter, would chemotherapy increase my chances of survival? What might happen to me because I'm not having it?

People who can't make decisions for themselves

While most older people will be able to make their own decisions, you may be reading this chapter because you are the relative of someone who has breast cancer and also suffers from a condition (such as memory loss, cognitive impairment or dementia) that affects their ability to understand what is happening and participate in decisions.

If your relative previously made arrangements for you to have something called 'Lasting Power of Attorney' (LPA) for Health and Welfare, you can make medical decisions on their behalf. If the LPA is just for Property and Financial Affairs, you cannot make medical decisions for them, and you cannot accept or refuse treatment on their behalf. If you don't have LPA, the doctors will still listen to your thoughts and wishes, but they will make the final medical decisions that they think are in the best interests of the patient. Macmillan's website has a useful section on cancer and dementia.

CHAPTER 23

SECONDARY (METASTATIC) BREAST CANCER

SECONDARY BREAST CANCER means that cancer cells have spread into your lymphatic or blood vessels and started to grow in a different part of your body. This new growth is called a 'metastasis' or 'met' for short. The most common sites for mets are your bones, lungs, liver and brain. Secondary breast cancer is also known as metastatic cancer, advanced cancer, recurrent cancer, Stage 4 cancer or distant spread. It cannot be cured, but it can be treated, and some patients live for many years after being diagnosed with it, although this depends on what metastases they have.

How common is secondary breast cancer?

Around 5 per cent of women with breast cancer have metastatic disease at the time of diagnosis. This is also called *de novo* metastatic disease. There is not a lot of accurate data about how many women with primary breast cancer get a recurrence, but the current estimate is that 20–30 per cent of women will get a recurrence in their lifetime. This does not mean that everyone has a 20–30 per cent chance of recurrence. Younger women are more likely to get a recurrence than older women, mainly because they are more likely to live long enough to get a recurrence. Also, women with a poor prognosis are more likely to get a recurrence than women with a good prognosis (see page 29).

If you have a high risk of recurrence when you are diagnosed, you are likely to be offered extra treatments such as chemotherapy and Herceptin (see Chapters 10 and 11) to reduce this risk. However, even if you have a slow-growing, low-risk cancer, it can still come back in 10 or 20 years' time.

Symptoms of secondary breast cancer

The symptoms of secondary breast cancer are often fairly vague and can mimic other medical conditions. Invasive ductal and lobular cancers (see Chapter 2) have different patterns of spread. Ductal cancer tends to spread to the bones, lymph nodes, lungs, liver and brain and is normally easily seen on scans. Lobular cancer, as well as spreading to the sites above, can also spread to your stomach, bowel and ovaries, and this can be much harder to see on a scan, simply because lobular cancer tends to grow in sheets of cells instead of forming a clump or mass. See page 270 for a useful infographic which summarises the symptoms of secondary breast cancer.

What is my prognosis?

Nobody wants to read this section. There is no easy way to come to terms with the fact that your cancer cannot be cured. How long you will live for depends on many things, including your age, whether your cancer is sensitive to oestrogen and Herceptin, and where in your body the metastases are. If you have only bone mets, you may live for many years with very few symptoms. If you have brain mets, however, your chances of living a long time are lower.

Your mets may have a different receptor status to your primary tumour, and they can even change receptor status over time. There is currently no way to predict how your cancer might respond to a certain treatment, and new treatments are always being developed. The aim of secondary breast cancer treatment is to try to keep it under control and stop it spreading further for as long as possible, often for many years. This means having treatment for the rest of your life.

TREATING SECONDARY BREAST CANCER

Everyone with secondary breast cancer is different. The treatment package that is best for *your* cancer will be worked out by your own cancer team, taking account of your needs and preferences. Your doctor will monitor you with blood tests for tumour markers (see page 28) and body scans. The treatments are often referred to as 'first-line', 'second-line' and 'third-line'. First-line treatments are the first drugs that your doctor will prescribe for you. If your cancer doesn't shrink or starts to grow, they will then try the second-line treatment, and so on. We can't cover all the individual treatments in detail in this chapter, but we want to give a brief overview of what is available. For more information and a social media link on the topics covered in this chapter, search online for 'METUP UK' – a campaign group committed to ending secondary breast cancer.

Most of the treatments for secondary breast cancer, such as chemotherapy, Herceptin and other targeted therapy, hormone therapy and bisphosphonates to strengthen your bones, are described in the earlier chapters in this book. You may be offered some or all of the above, depending on where your metastases are and what previous treatments you have had. In fact, many women who only have bone disease are just treated with hormone treatment and bisphosphonates, and do not need chemotherapy. In the next sections, we go into a bit more detail about some of the more specific treatments that you might need.

Surgery

If you only have a small amount of cancer in one organ or bone (also called *oligometastatic* disease) and it is easy to reach, your oncologist may recommend surgery to remove the metastatic deposit. Surgery can also be used for symptom control – for example, if you break a bone in your leg because it has been weakened by cancer, an orthopaedic surgeon can insert metal plates and screws to fix it.

Radiofrequency ablation

This is a technique that uses heat to destroy cancer deposits in organs like your liver. It can be done under sedation or with a general anaesthetic. Using ultrasound or CT guidance, fine needles with electrodes on the ends are inserted into the tumour, and these electrodes heat the tumour with the aim of destroying it.

Radiotherapy

Radiotherapy is given for pain control and to slow down spread, and is often used to treat your bones, your brain or your skin. You normally only have a couple of treatments instead of the long course given to the breast for primary cancer. If you have only one or two small areas of cancer in one organ, such as your brain, you may be given stereotactic radiotherapy (also called 'Gammaknife' or 'Cyberknife', after the machines that are used). This involves a very high dose of radiotherapy treatment which accurately targets the metastatic area, and may only be available in larger, specialist cancer hospitals.

Drains

If you have cancer in your lungs or liver, it can cause fluid to build up around your lungs or in your tummy. This can make it difficult to breathe, or your tummy might swell and feel very uncomfortable. You might need to have this fluid drained to make things easier. This can be done as a one-off procedure, or your doctors may leave a permanent drain inside your chest or tummy so the fluid keeps draining away (see page 128).

Treatment as part of a research trial

Sadly, most research on breast cancer to date has focused on primary breast cancer. Partly as a result of pressure from patients with secondary breast cancer, more research is starting to focus on how to prevent and treat it. Cancer Research UK has a list of all the current trials for breast cancer (see Chapter 6 for more on research trials), and this is a good place to start if you want to look for a trial that might suit you. It is important to look for trials sooner rather than later, as you may become ineligible to join a trial if you have already had certain treatments first. You may also need to travel to a larger cancer centre to take part in the trial, and the travel, on top of the side effects of treatment, can be taxing on you and your family.

QUESTIONS TO ASK YOUR DOCTOR

The following questions might help you decide what treatment to have:

- How extensive are my mets? Is only part of my body involved or several? If there is only one, can it be removed with surgery or radiotherapy?
- What is my cancer's receptor status (i.e. is it ER+ve and/ or HER2+ve)? Is this different from my primary tumour?
- Am I well enough to tolerate stronger treatments such as chemotherapy and surgery if I need them? How often will I need them and how will they make me feel?
- How will my treatment affect my quality of life? Can I carry on working? (You need to decide whether you are prepared to put up with certain side effects even if these lower your quality of life.)
- How will I be monitored? What scans and tests will I need and how will you know if the treatments are working?
- Are there any research trials that I can take part in?
- What happens when the treatments stop working?

It can be very hard deciding what treatment to have, and how much to have. there is always a trade-off between possible benefits of a treatment and potential side effects. if your cancer starts to grow despite switching treatments, or the drugs are making you feel rotten all the time, you may need to think about a gentler but less effective treatment or stopping treatment altogether.

LIVING WITH SECONDARY BREAST CANCER

Whereas Trish and Liz wrote most of this book from personal experience, they haven't had personal experience of metastatic disease. Below, we quote, with kind permission, from 'After Breast Cancer Diagnosis', the website of Jo Taylor, a patient advocate with Stage 4 breast cancer herself:

In February 2014 I was diagnosed with secondary breast cancer. As like my primary breast cancer diagnosis, it was a huge shock. Many people don't understand secondary breast cancer or that it doesn't actually come back in your breast. That would be classed as a local recurrence or another primary breast cancer. Mine came back in my lymph nodes in my neck and I ended up with a couple of small spots in my sternum.

In a way, I was lucky not to have any of the major organs affected. But yet it's still hard to comprehend and come to terms with, yet life carries on. I hope that it can be controlled and that it doesn't progress further for a while.

I have treatment every 3 weeks for life, forever. I will have to continue this treatment otherwise the cancer will return and spread so that's why you have to continue with the regime. The treatments hope to control the cancer. Again people don't understand this, yes I may have hair on my head and be able to exercise but I have an incurable disease and that's why I have to continue going to [hospital] every 3 weeks.

I have my bad days, days when I get a migraine from the treatment and I cannot function, aches and pains due to the drugs that I'm on, pain from the peripheral neuropathy in my toes and fingers but currently I'm doing OK.

One of the challenges of coping with secondary breast cancer is the uncertainty around the question 'How long have I got?'. No doctor can give you an accurate estimate as everybody responds differently to treatment, and new treatments are being developed all the time.

Macmillan and Breast Cancer Care have separate sections for patients with secondary breast cancer, and you can get a lot of information and support from these websites. The US-based National Breast Cancer Foundation also has a lot of helpful information. (See pages 277–81 for further details of these organisations.)

One of the best ways to cope with secondary breast cancer is to link up with others who are going through it – either online (such as through the forums on the Macmillan and Breast Cancer Care websites) or in a support group. There are also many breast cancer bloggers who write eloquently about living with secondary cancer, such as 'Stickit2stage4'. You could also try blogging yourself. This can be a good way of dealing with your emotions, interacting with others and letting friends and family know what is going on. Social media, such as Twitter and Facebook, can also be an excellent resource for support, advice and information.

It can really help to read what other patients have gone through, and to know that you're not alone. There are several breast cancer memoirs that can be quite harrowing to read, especially as most of them end with the woman eventually dying due to cancer. For a more positive take, we strongly recommend *Metastatic Madness: How I Coped With A Stage 4 Cancer Diagnosis* (XLIBRIS, 2012) by Carol Miele, a nurse with secondary breast cancer. It's well-written, funny, personal and – believe it or not – hopeful.

Palliative care

'Palliate' means 'to relieve or make better'. It's not the same as terminal care, which is only for the dying. The distinction is important, because you may benefit from so-called palliative care long before you are terminally ill. Palliative care is usually coordinated through liaison between your oncology team, your GP and specialist palliative care professionals, notably Macmillan nurses. If you are terminally ill, a hospice may be involved.

Palliative care consists of a number of things, including:

- Emotional and practical support from people who are used to working with those who have secondary cancer, to help you cope and optimise your quality of life.
- Adjusting drug doses to get the right balance between benefit and side effects.
- Help with pain control, including medication but also behavioural and cognitive approaches, as well as physical ones, such as TENS machines.
- Help with nausea, including careful review of your medication and advice on your diet and lifestyle.
- Help with other ongoing symptoms, such as constipation, skin sores, and so on.
- Emergency help if you deteriorate.
- Helping families come to terms with your diagnosis and understand how they can support you.
- Helping with end-of-life planning (see below).

Different localities have different arrangements for palliative care. If in doubt, ask your oncology nurse or GP.

Planning for the end of your life

If you're reading this section, you have either reached the stage that there are no treatments left and your cancer is progressing, or you're curious to know what the worst-case scenario is, even if you're not there yet. None of this is easy, but it is important to think, talk and plan about where you want to die, and make sure your doctors and family are aware of your wishes.

The finality of knowing that you are going to die soon can make you feel fear, anxiety, anger, hopelessness, guilt, loneliness, depression and grief. Add to this worrying about what will happen to your family when you have gone can be incredibly overwhelming. We cannot even pretend to understand what this is like. However, we have both watched close friends die from cancer, and seen the different ways in which they coped.

Some patients have said that facing up to the reality of death, planning for it and talking to family and doctors about it can help with negative emotions. You may sleep easier and be able to take one day at a time if you have a plan for your own end-of-life and have begun to settle your affairs. This isn't giving up; it's getting real. Taking some control back may bring you a sense of relief and even peace. Indeed, you may find that you are better able to face reality than some of your loved ones.

Some people have a bucket list of things they want to do before they die, but if you suddenly become too ill to complete it, this could make you feel worse. Instead, you might want to create something enduring for your loved ones (perhaps in the form of a 'memory box' of photos and your favourite things, letters to be opened on future birthdays, or a book or blog). You may have a project you want to finish – or hand on – before you die.

You should almost certainly make a will, sort out your financial affairs and pull together documents your partner or family will need after your death (such as passwords to any accounts you'd like them to be able to access, and your life insurance details, if relevant). If you have young children or pets, you should think about making plans for how they will be looked after when you die. You may wish to give your partner Lasting Power of Attorney especially if there is a possibility that you may lose your ability to make your own decisions. An advance directive ('living will') is also a good idea. Macmillan call this an Advance Decision to Refuse Treatment and cover it in the 'Sorting Things Out' section on their website (www.macmillan.org.uk). You may also want to think about your funeral. This is never going to be easy, but you might want to talk about this with your loved ones so they know what you would like when the inevitable happens. Do you have a favourite song that you want to be played, or want everyone to wear your favourite colour? Instead of people sending flowers, you may want to ask them to donate to a cause close to your heart.

Death and dying remains a taboo subject in our society. The excellent charity Dying Matters (www.dyingmatters.org) offers more information for the dying and their loved ones, and also campaigns for more openness about death and dying. Another excellent website is Compassion in Dying (https://compassionin-dying.org.uk).

Coping with a diagnosis of secondary breast cancer must be incredibly difficult, and neither of us can imagine what you are going through. We do want you to know that you don't need to stay positive all the time, and that it is okay to swear and shout and cry if it helps. Although your diagnosis may seem like a death sentence at the time, there are many women who still live a fulfilling and active life in between their regular treatments, and outlive their predicted survival. There is also a large online community of women who are constantly pushing for more research into metastatic cancer, and we live in hope that one day a drug will be developed that will cure breast cancer.

CHAPTER 24

MOVING FORWARD

ONCE YOU HAVE finished all your hospital treatments, friends and family may expect you to go back to normal, as you are now 'cancer-free'. However, we found that this period is often harder to deal with than the treatments themselves, especially as you are no longer seen regularly in the hospital, and are living with the fear of recurrence.

HOW WILL YOU BE FOLLOWED UP?

Breast cancer follow-up care anywhere in the UK, whether NHS or private, follows evidence-based National Institute for Health and Care Excellence guidelines (see Chapter 6). These recommend that you should have an agreed care plan, with joint care between your cancer team and your GP.

Hospital follow-up

In the UK, everyone should be seen by a doctor or a breast care nurse at one year after diagnosis, and again at five years. If you have had chemotherapy or been involved in a clinical trial, you may also be seen regularly by your oncology team over the first five years. Your doctor will examine you to look for signs of recurrence. If you aren't happy with the appearance of your breasts, now is a good time to discuss with your surgeon whether another operation might be able to improve things. They will ask you how you are coping with the side effects of your treatment, such as hormone therapy, and discuss how long you should keep taking it for. They may also do a holistic assessment, where they ask about all the other parts of your life that can be affected by cancer, such as money, relationship issues and your mood. The results of this assessment will be fed back to your GP, along with an agreed action plan.

Seeing your GP

Your GP will not invite you for a check-up. However, as an NHS patient, you can go to your GP at any time if you need medication, are worried about a symptom or simply feel you're not coping. Your GP probably knew you before you got cancer, and will want to share your joy and relief after treatment ends. He or she can supply you with sick notes if you're not ready to return to work, and will be well placed to support you if you're not coping emotionally. If you're nervous about seeing your GP (for example, if you don't know them well), make a list of the things you want to discuss and put the most important ones at the top. GP surgeries usually have practice nurses who offer appointments, and you may find the nurse has more time for you and is more approachable.

Screening mammograms

If you still have a breast on the other side, you will have yearly mammograms for five years. When they finish, if you are over 50 you will go into the NHS Breast Screening Programme and be invited for mammograms every three years. If you are under 50, you will continue to have mammograms every year until you enter the Screening Programme. If you are over 70 and are no longer routinely invited for screening mammograms, you can self-refer for a mammogram every three years.

If you had dense breasts when you were diagnosed or your cancer wasn't seen on a mammogram, research has shown that mammograms are still the most effective way of screening your other breast, because most new breast cancers are easy to see on a mammogram. Your breasts normally become less dense with hormone therapy and the effects of the menopause. If your breasts are still dense or your mammogram is hard to interpret, your doctor may then recommend an MRI.

In between hospital appointments

Most breast units in the UK offer open-access follow-up or are moving towards that option. This means you can phone up the breast care nurse if you have a problem and she will arrange for you to be seen in clinic. This is often quicker than going to see your GP and getting a new referral, though you may prefer to do it that way. In sum, if you have a problem between your booked appointments, you have two choices: see your GP or call your breast care nurse.

HOW WILL YOU KNOW IF YOUR CANCER HAS COME BACK?

There are two ways that breast cancer can come back – either as a local recurrence in the breast tissue, skin or axillary lymph nodes, or as a distant recurrence in your bones or organs. Distant recurrence is the same as secondary breast cancer (see Chapter 23). When you have finished treatment, you should be told what the signs and symptoms of local and distant recurrence are. Breast Cancer Care have a good leaflet that explains this in more detail. It is effectively up to you to police yourself and to learn what is normal and not for you.

Local recurrence

The symptoms of a local recurrence are similar to the symptoms of primary cancer (see Chapter 2) or can show as a lump in or near your scar. You may also notice a red raised area like a spot or an ulcer if the cancer comes back in your skin. However, surgery and radiotherapy can make your breast feel hard or lumpy, and it can be hard to know what is normal after treatment. If you have any concerns, ask your GP to refer you back to the breast clinic. Local recurrence is normally treated with surgery first (see Chapter 7).

Distant recurrence

The symptoms of distance recurrence (secondary breast cancer) are explained on page 270. Jo Taylor, a patient advocate with Stage 4 breast cancer, produced this excellent infographic (see page 270) which summarises the symptoms of secondary breast cancer:

If you have any of these symptoms, see your GP or call your breast care nurse and ask to be seen quickly. We know from experience that in the first few months and even years after treatment, every little twinge is anxiety-provoking. Your symptoms may have a simple explanation, but your doctor will probably arrange some tests to make sure. We cover the treatment of secondary breast cancer in Chapter 23.

COPING WITH THE 'NEW NORMAL'

While you are having breast cancer treatment, you have a lot of hospital visits, appointments and tests. Once you have finished treatment, this all stops. Understandably, after all the attention and emotional trauma of the initial treatment phase, it is common to feel abandoned and anxious rather than relieved or exhilarated when your doctor waves you goodbye and says, 'See you in four years.' This is the time when you really start to come to terms with your cancer diagnosis, and what living with cancer is actually like. You probably have lots of questions, such as:

- Am I the only person who feels like this?
- Who is going to check up on me?
- How will I cope at home and at work?
- Where can I get support?

Secondary Breast Cancer

Also known as metastatic or advanced breast cancer

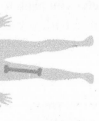

If you have survived primary breast cancer be aware of these **RED flags***
for secondary breast cancer. There are 5 main areas that secondary
breast cancer can appear.

BRAIN

Frequent headaches, vomiting
(first thing in the am), dizzy, visual
disturbance, fits, impaired
intellectual function, mood
swings, balance, fatigue. Family
members and friends may say
you are not your normal self.

BONE

Pain in bones — commonly
thigh, arm, ribs and back. Can be
dull ache or sharp shooting
pain. Bone pain with no obvious
cause or haven't fallen over,
report any new, unusual and
increasing pain.

LYMPH NODES

Swelling or lumps and
pressure in chest/armpit/
neck areas, dry cough.

LUNG

Sharp pain on breathing in
chest and back area, non
productive cough, fatigue,
blood clots can also cause
shortness of breath.

LIVER

Bloating, affected appetite,
weight loss, fatigue, weak,
pain near ribs on right
hand side.

*RED FLAG SYMPTOMS NEED TO BE REPORTED TO YOUR ONCOLOGIST

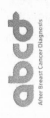

abcd

After Breast Cancer Diagnosis

Please visit: abcdiagnosis.co.uk
Twitter: @abcdiagnosis
Facebook: facebook.com/abcdiagnosis

There are no rules about what you should or should not feel. A survey of 800 breast cancer survivors by the charity Breast Cancer Care found that just over half of people with breast cancer struggled with anxiety after the end of treatment. More than a quarter described life after the illness as 'tougher than the illness itself', and nearly one-third had symptoms of depression (e.g. overwhelming sadness, tearfulness or difficulty seeing the positive side in anything). Anxiety can be particularly bad when you're coming up to your next check-up ('scanxiety'). The stress of waiting to find out your scan results can be unbearable.

The Breast Cancer Care survey identified three top issues for women immediately after completing treatment for breast cancer: fear of the cancer coming back (80 per cent), fatigue (79 per cent) and lack of body confidence (52 per cent). Only 1 in 10 of women felt 'positive and ready to move on'. Indeed, some breast cancer survivors use the term 'collateral damage' to refer to the knock-on (and sometimes permanent) effects that cancer has on their body, self-esteem, relationship, job, and so on.

Dr Peter Harvey, a cancer psychologist, has written a very useful summary of the emotional and physical roller coaster of cancer treatment called 'After the treatment finishes – then what?':

It is a widely-held belief ... that the treatment of an illness is meant to make you feel better. One of the many paradoxes of cancer is that, more often than not, the treatment makes you feel worse. This is not surprising – we cut and possibly mutilate, inject you with poisonous and powerful chemicals, subject you to dangerous rays all in the name of treatment. The aggressiveness and power of the treatments are a necessary response to the power of the disease, of course, but this very power takes its toll in other ways. These interventions place enormous physical strains on the body. There is often little time to recover from one treatment before the next one starts. The treatments themselves may make it difficult for you to sleep and eat properly – two important parts of the body's defence and recovery system. Some of the treatments drain your energy and resources to such an extent that it's as much as you can do to put on the kettle. Add to this the emotional turmoil – the dealing with the impact and implications of the diagnosis, the uncertainty, the upheaval, the additional burden that you feel that you are imposing on family and friends, the loss of so many aspects of your routine. Emotional stress can be as energy consuming as any physical activity. After all that, is it any wonder that you feel wrung out and exhausted, without resources or reserves?

Don't be too hard on yourself if you don't feel as good on the inside as you look on the outside. Your physical symptoms will gradually settle down over the next couple of months, but the emotional side effects – the fear of your cancer returning, waking up each day wondering if this is the day it comes back, worrying whether your winter cold is actually a recurrence – can take years to resolve. All of these thoughts and feelings do get better in time (trust us – we've been there). However, it may be hard for your friends and loved ones to understand your turmoil. In their eyes you don't have cancer any more, and life should return to normal.

It may help to stop thinking about getting 'back to normal' (that is, returning to exactly the same state you were in before you got cancer) and instead think about 'adjusting to a new normal'. Let's face it – life has a different meaning now, doesn't it? Some things have become unimportant. Some things have gone forever. Other things have endured and even strengthened. Your 'new normal' can include, for example:

- New and different friendships.
- A different body image (that takes time to learn to love).
- Difficulty doing things you used to do, both physically and mentally.
- Emotional scars from the trauma of treatment.
- A different relationship with your partner and/or children.
- A different attitude towards your job.
- Accepting that you are unable to have children.

You may not like your 'new normal' as much as the life you had before cancer. You may grieve the body you had (or even the marriage you had) before cancer came along. As hard as this is, you can't turn back the clock. Life goes on. It just takes time to adjust, and some people need a lot longer than others.

Make sure you look after yourself. As we said in Chapter 18, eat a healthy diet and do some regular exercise, especially as these can both reduce the risk of recurrence. Find ways to relax, either alone or with others. If you think that a more structured programme of group support is what you need right now, sign up for one of the 'Moving Forward' courses offered by Breast Cancer Care. These usually run for half a day a week for four weeks. They offer factual information but also a strong and positive group psychology for tackling the next stage in your life.

Post-traumatic stress disorder

While symptoms of moderate anxiety and depression are common during breast cancer treatment and in the immediate aftermath (see page 41), they usually lessen as the months go by. Rarely, people can develop post-traumatic stress disorder (PTSD) – sometimes months or years after their cancer treatment. An excellent account of PTSD (and some good tips on how to cope with it) can be found on Steve Pake's blog. Steve had a different cancer but his insights about PTSD are applicable to breast cancer:

> I arrived at work on a seemingly ordinary day on Thursday, May 21st, but found myself unable to think or concentrate at all. I felt a lot of nervous energy and anxiety building, but didn't know why. I had also started having cancer-related nightmares in the previous week, as if to predict something rotten coming. It turned out that this particular day was my last two days of chemotherapy, four years ago, and I remember those days all too well. I was so afraid that the chemo wasn't going to work, wondering if I was still going to die or not, and I was tired of being poisoned almost to death and feeling like complete hell. The only thing that stopped me

273

from ripping off my lines and running away were an extra few doses of [a relaxant drug], and its induced haze and false calm. All of these fears and emotions had been buried, but here they were, suddenly coming to the surface four years later. I was right back in that oncology infusion room again as if it were happening now, and I was absolutely terrified. I went to a quiet and secluded corner at my office where nobody was likely to find me, and there I sat with hands trembling and my head between my knees as the tears started falling.

People say to just not think about these things, but they don't realize that I'm <u>not</u> thinking about them, consciously at least. It's from our sub-conscious. <u>It's</u> thinking about it, and causing us to re-experience these memories as if they were happening on that very day. The same powerful emotions of extreme fear, that fight-or-flight adrenaline, and the instinct to run away, right now, came out.

If this sounds like what you're going through, you should seek professional help. PTSD is very distressing but it is often very treatable (for example with cognitive behavioural therapy). See your GP or mention it to your oncology team.

GIVING SOMETHING BACK

A lot of people feel grateful for all the care and attention they have received and want to give something back to help others. This may be as simple as donating money to your local breast unit or taking part in a sporting challenge to raise money for a cancer charity like Macmillan, Breast Cancer Care or Breast Cancer Now. There are also lots of small events all over the UK such as the popular 'Race for Life', and it can be great fun to go along with your family and friends, dressed in pink from head to toe. It may also give you a new-found appreciation for your body; what it is capable of dealing with and what it can do for you now. Look after it – you only have one.

We did a 100km women-only bike ride through the night to raise money for women's cancer charities, wearing pink feather boas and tutus. It was amazing to be surrounded by thousands of women affected by cancer. We raised over £2,000 between us, and the event as a whole raised over £1 million in one night.

Being diagnosed with breast cancer is life-changing – not just for you, but for your family and friends as well. It can feel like you're on a roller coaster with no way of controlling what's happening to you, but it's not all negative. Although our lives are completely different now, in a small way, they are better than they were before. We have made so many new friends, we appreciate just what our bodies can to do for us, and we have learned that spending time with our loved ones is what gets us through each day. We hope that we've empowered you to understand what is happening to you, and given you the strength to cope.

RESOURCES

We reproduce the links to websites below in good faith but we don't endorse everything they say.

Websites

Adoption UK
www.adoptionuk.org

Adjuvant! Online
www.newadjuvant.com/default2.aspx

After Breast Cancer Diagnosis
www.abcdiagnosis.co.uk

American Society of Clinical Oncology
www.asco.org

Amoena
www.amoena.com/uk-en

Association of Breast Surgery
https://associationofbreastsurgery.org.uk

The Big C
www.big-c.co.uk

BreastCancer.org
https://community.breastcancer.org

Breast Cancer Care
www.breastcancercare.org.uk

Artistic tattoos
www.breastcancercare.org.uk/information-support/facing-breast-cancer/living-beyond-breast-cancer/your-body/your-body-after-breast-cancer-treatment/artistic-tattoos-after-breast-cancer-surgery

Breast cancer in men
www.breastcancercare.org.uk/information-support/have-i-got-breast-cancer/breast-cancer-in-men

Breast cancer stages
www.breastcancercare.org.uk/information-support/facing-breast-cancer/diagnosed-breast-cancer/diagnosis/breast-cancer-stages

Breast reconstruction guide
www.breastcancercare.org.uk/information-support/facing-breast-cancer/going-through-treatment-breast-cancer/surgery/breast-7

Moving forward
www.breastcancercare.org.uk/information-support/support-you/local-support/moving-forward-after-breast-cancer-treatment

Recipes from the Royal Marsden Cookbook
www.breastcancercare.org.uk/information-support/vita-magazine/recipes-royal-marsden-cancer-cookbook

Someone like me
www.breastcancercare.org.uk/information-support/support-you/someone-talk/someone-me

Your body after breast cancer treatment
www.breastcancercare.org.uk/information-support/facing-breast-cancer/living-beyond-breast-cancer/your-body/your-body-after-breast-cancer-treatment

Worries about breast cancer coming back
www.breastcancercare.org.uk/information-support/facing-breast-cancer/living-beyond-breast-cancer/coping-emotionally/worries-about-breast-cancer-coming-back

Breast Cancer Haven
www.breastcancerhaven.org.uk

Breast Cancer Now
www.breastcancernow.org

British Association for Behavioural & Cognitive Psychotherapies
www.babcp.com

British Cycling breeze rides
www.letsride.co.uk/breeze

Cancer Fit
www.cancerfit.me

Cancer Research UK
www.cancerresearchuk.org

Find a clinical trial
www.cancerresearchuk.org/about-cancer/find-a-clinical-trial

CaringBridge
www.caringbridge.org

Cathy Leman
www.dammadaboutbreastcancer.com

Chai Cancer Care
www.chaicancercare.org

Childlessness Overcome Through Surrogacy (COTS)
www.surrogacy.org.uk

Clinical Trials Explained
http://clinicaltrialsexplained.com

Compassion in Dying
https://compassionindying.org.uk

Making decisions and planning your care
https://compassionindying.org.uk/making-decisions-and-planning-your-care

Coram BAAF Adoption and Fostering Academy
https://corambaaf.org.uk

The Daisy Network
www.daisynetwork.org.uk

Dietitian UK
www.dietitianuk.co.uk

Dream Challenges Ride the Night
www.dream-challenges.com/challenges/women-v-cancer/ride-the-night/

Dying Matters
www.dyingmatters.org

Eek!! My Mummy Has Breast Cancer
www.eekmymummy.co.uk

Free Spirit
www.freespirittravelinsurance.com

Headspace
www.headspace.com

Human Fertilisation & Embryology Authority
www.hfea.gov.uk

Inspire
www.inspire.com

Insurancewith
www.insurancewith.com

Knitted Knockers UK
www.kkukciowix.com

Live Better With Cancer
www.livebetterwith.com

Macmillan
www.macmillan.org.uk

Finding the words
www.macmillan.org.uk/_images/Finding%20the%20words_
tcm9-313290.pdf

Mobile app
www.macmillan.org.uk/yourmacnews/archives/winter2014/
features/myorganiser.aspx

Macom
www.macom-medical.com/post-surgery/bras

Maggie's
www.maggiescentres.org

METUP.org
http://metup.org

MIND
www.mind.org.uk

MSK Cancer Centre
www.mskcc.org

Mummy's Star
www.mummysstar.org

National Breast Cancer Foundation
www.nationalbreastcancer.org

Stage 4 breast cancer
www.nationalbreastcancer.org/breast-cancer-stage-4

National Institute for Health and Care Excellence
www.nice.org.uk

NHS Choices
www.nhs.uk/pages/home.aspx

Nicola Jane
www.nicolajane.com

Penny Brohn UK
www.pennybrohn.org.uk

P.ink
www.p-ink.org

PREDICT
www.predict.nhs.uk

RecoHeart
www.recoheart.com

Stress No More
www.stressnomore.co.uk

Touch Surgery
www.touchsurgery.com

WordPress
https://wordpress.com

Working With Cancer
www.workingwithcancer.co.uk

World Cancer Research Fund: 'Eating well during cancer'
www.wcrf-uk.org/uk/recipes/eat-well-during-cancer

World First
www.world-first.co.uk

Yes: the Organic Intimacy Company
www.yesyesyes.org

Blogs and Videos

Cancer Answers, MD
http://canceranswersmd.com

Here Comes the Sun
www.herecomesthesun927.com

The Jar of Joy TEDx talk
www.youtube.com/watch?v=Wc1PIAG8Bgg

Lisa Bonchek Adams
www.lisabadams.com

The small c
www.thesmallc.com

Stickit2Stage 4
https://stickit2stage4.com

Young Adult Cancer Survivorship by Steve Pake: PTSD After Cancer
www.stevepake.com/ptsd-after-cancer

Books, Articles and Downloads

Bartley, T., *Mindfulness: A Kindly Approach to Being with Cancer* (Wiley-Blackwell, 2016)

Cancer Council, 'Talking to Kids about Cancer' (2015), www.cancervic.org.au/downloads/resources/booklets/talking-to-kids-about-cancer/Talking-to-Kids-About-Cancer.pdf

Forrest, G., *Mummy's Lump*, Breast Cancer Care (2015), www.breastcancercare.org.uk/sites/default/files/publications/pdf/mummys_lump_2015_web.pdf

Greenhalgh, T., *How to Read a Paper: The basics of evidence-based medicine* (John Wiley & Sons, 2014. New edition forthcoming 2019)

Harvey, P., 'After the Treatment Finishes – Then What?', www.peterboroughbreastcancersupportgroup.co.uk/images/pdfs/AfterTreatment.pdf

Miele, C., *Metastatic Madness: How I Coped With A Stage 4 Cancer Diagnosis* (XLIBRIS, 2012)

Saez, L., 'Cancer and the Snake Oil Industry', *Huffington Post* (17 April 2017), www.huffingtonpost.co.uk/lawrence-saez/cancer-and-the-snake-oil-_b_16056342.html

Shaw, C., *The Royal Marsden Cancer Cookbook* (Kyle Books, 2015)

INDEX